AF598108

Diseases of Pleura

Edited by Jelena Stojšić

Published in London, United Kingdom

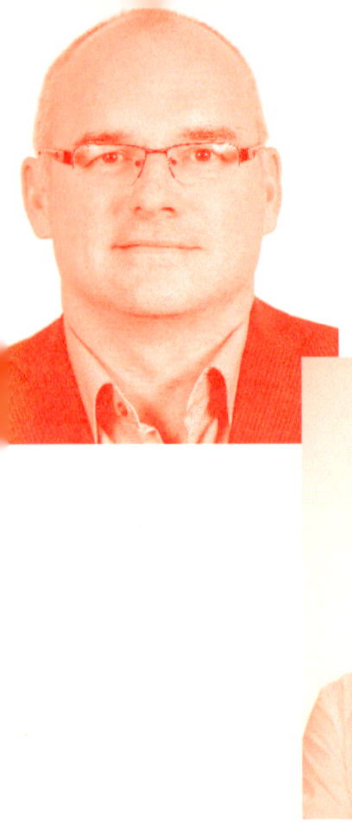
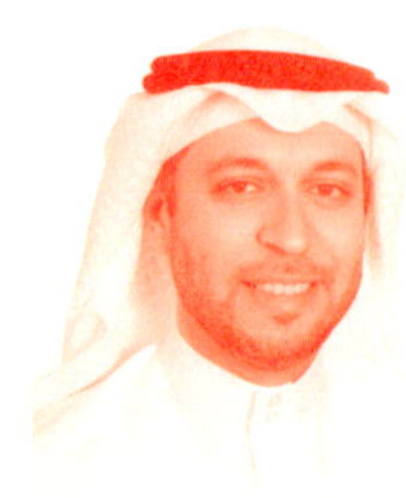
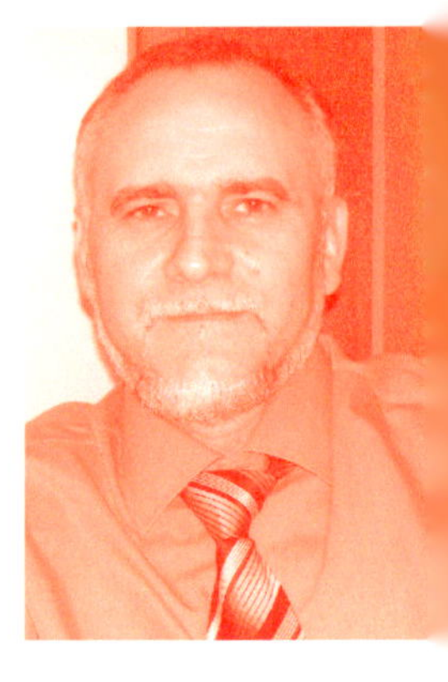
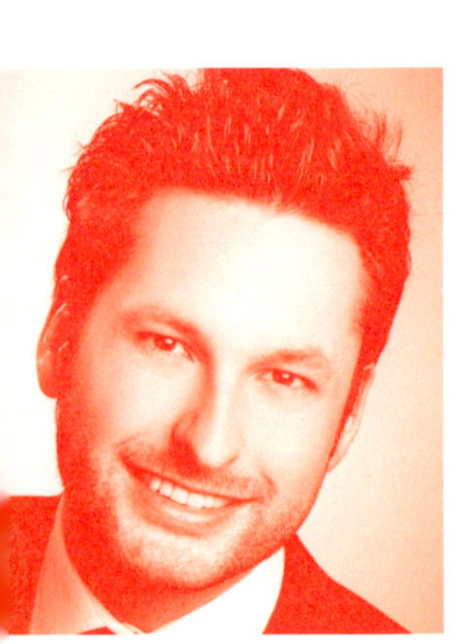
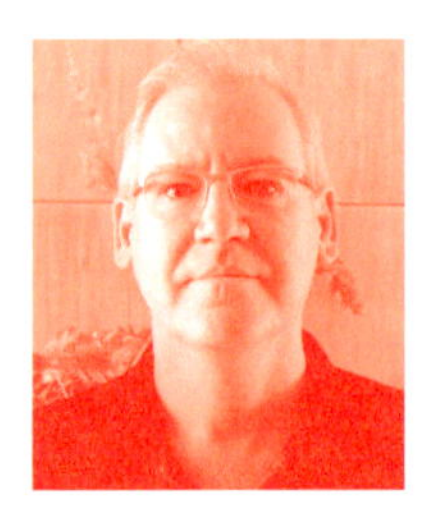
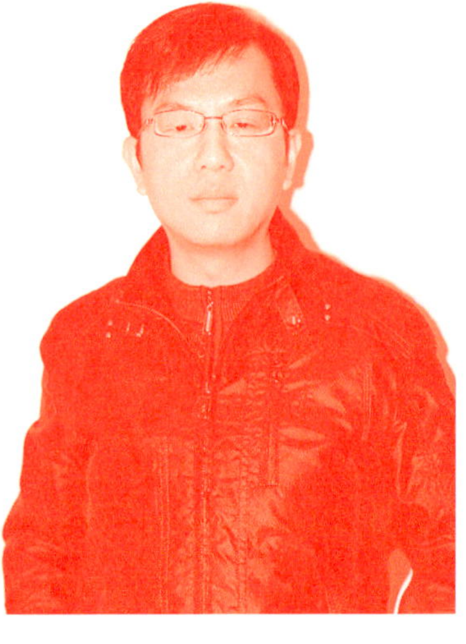

IntechOpen

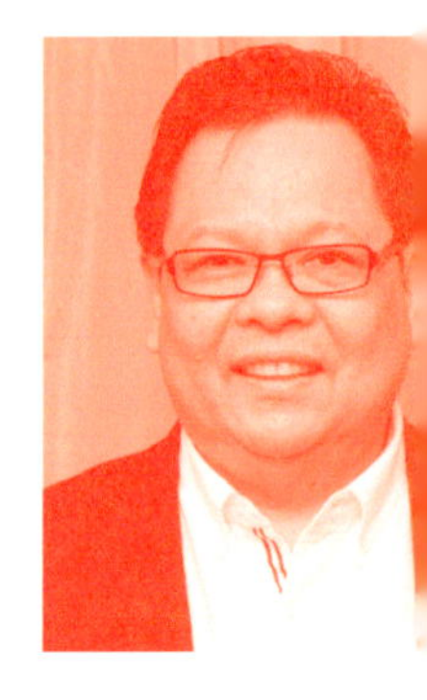
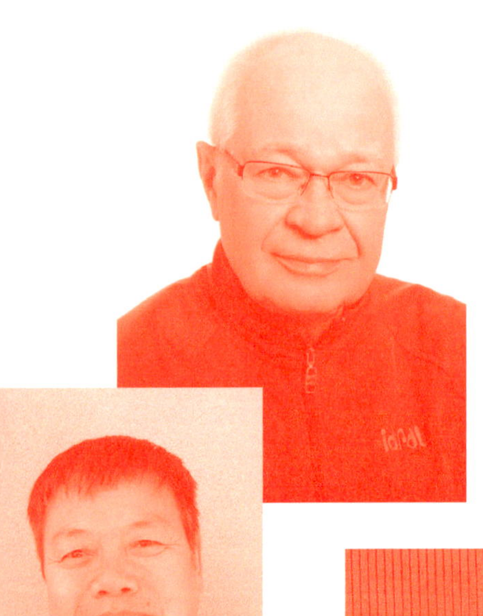
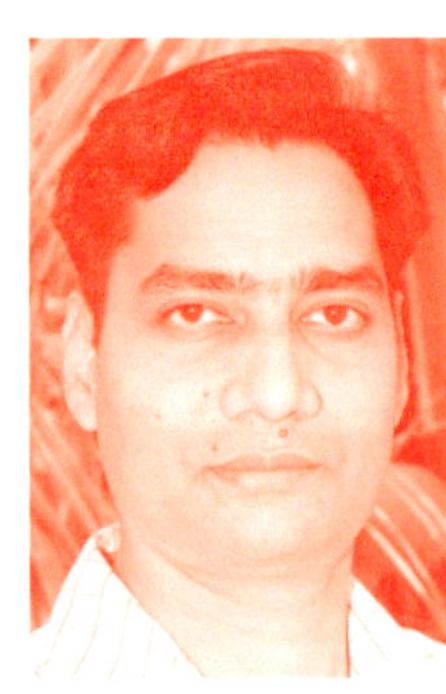
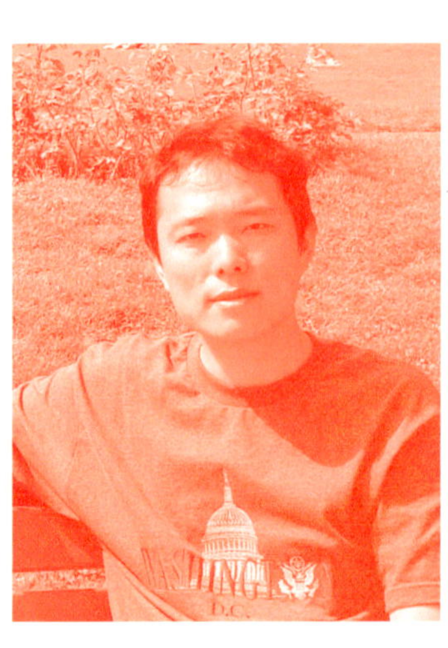
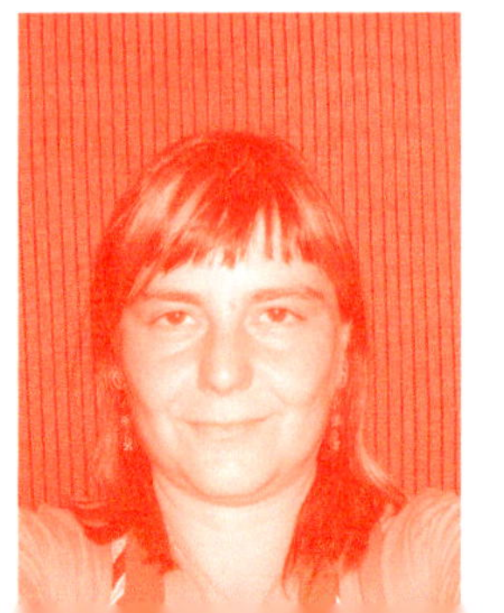

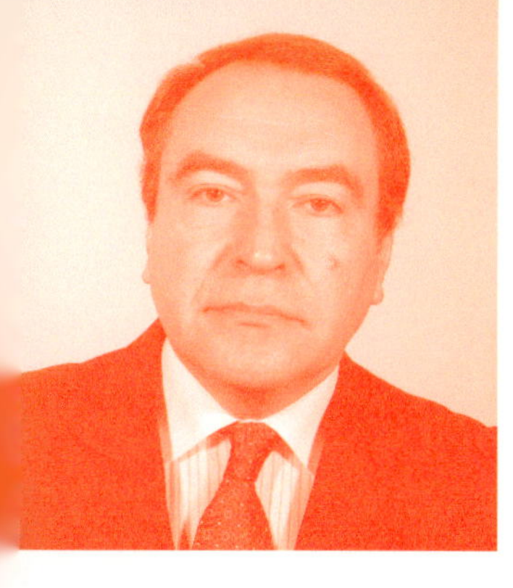

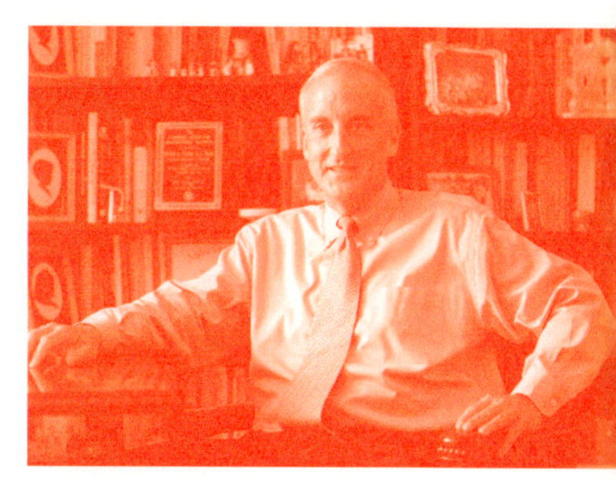

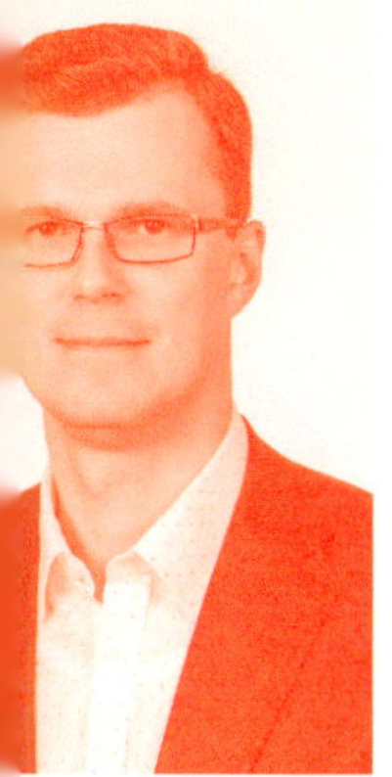

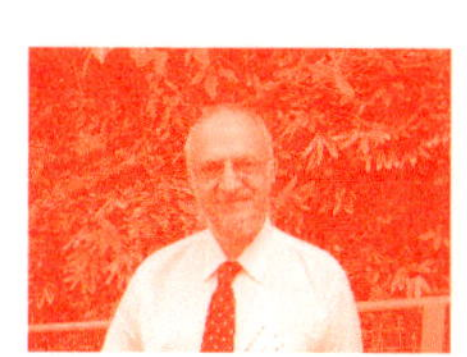

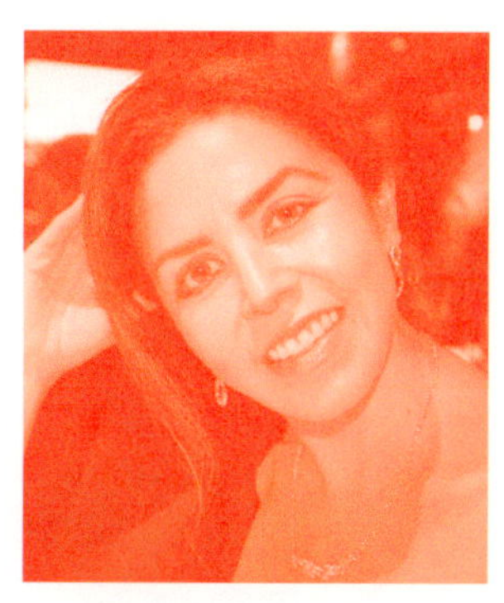

Supporting open minds since 2005

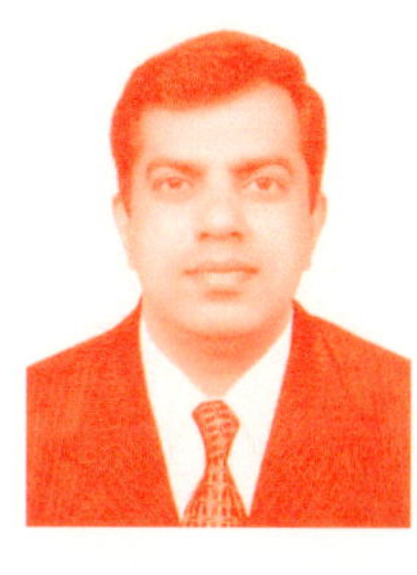

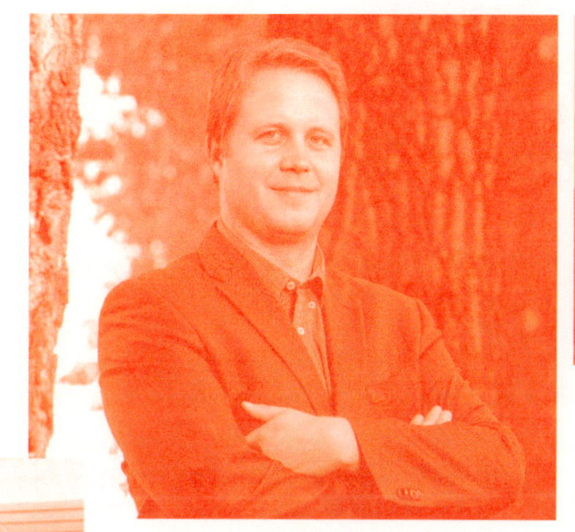

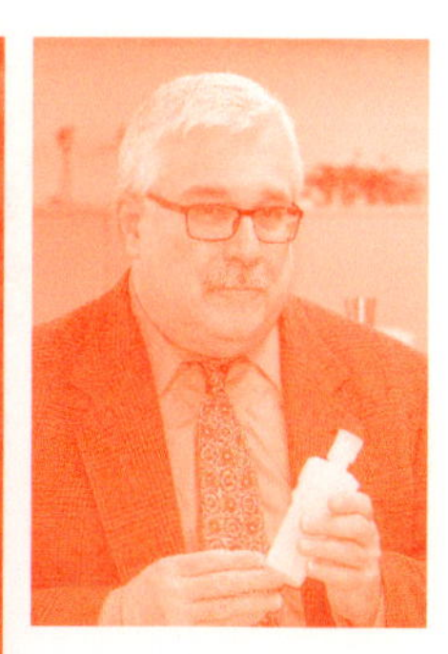

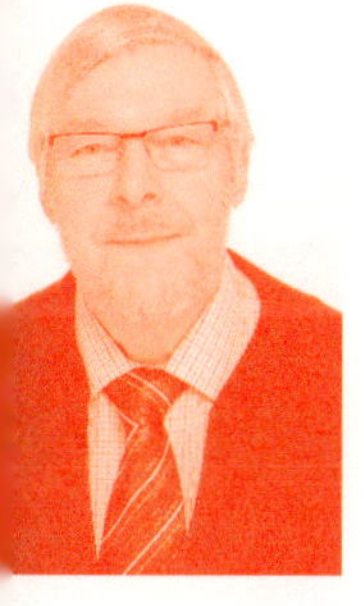

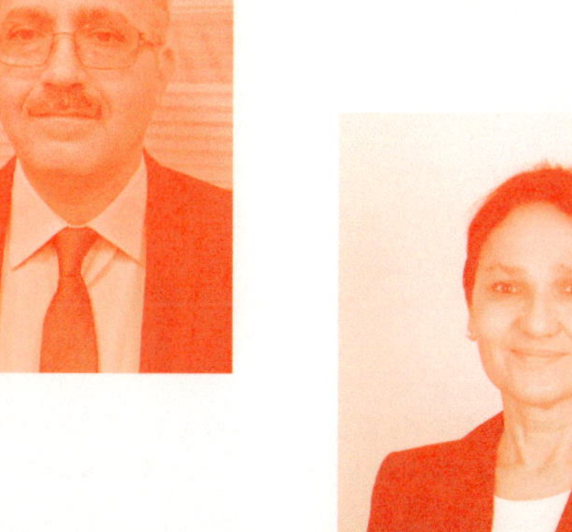

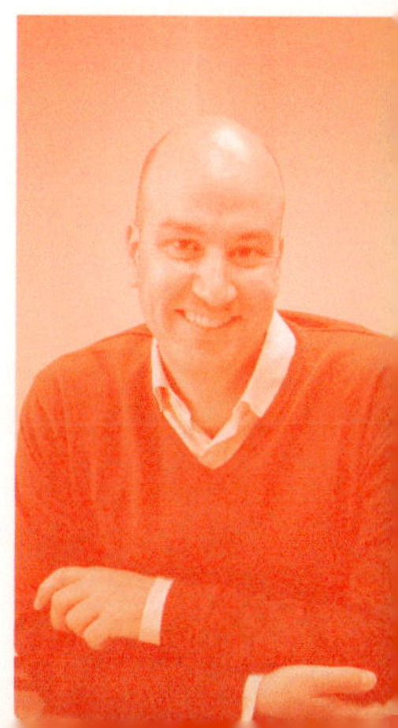

Diseases of Pleura
http://dx.doi.org/10.5772/intechopen.73954
Edited by Jelena Stojšić

Contributors
Alberto Sandri, Alessandro Maraschi, Matteo Gagliasso, Carlotta Cartia, Federica Massa, Luisella Righi, Francesco Ardissone, Roberta Rapanà, Simona Sobrero, Guntug Batihan, Kenan Ceylan, Ronald Gordon, Vita Dolžan, Alenka Franko, Jelena Stojšić

© The Editor(s) and the Author(s) 2020
The rights of the editor(s) and the author(s) have been asserted in accordance with the Copyright, Designs and Patents Act 1988. All rights to the book as a whole are reserved by INTECHOPEN LIMITED. The book as a whole (compilation) cannot be reproduced, distributed or used for commercial or non-commercial purposes without INTECHOPEN LIMITED's written permission. Enquiries concerning the use of the book should be directed to INTECHOPEN LIMITED rights and permissions department (permissions@intechopen.com).
Violations are liable to prosecution under the governing Copyright Law.

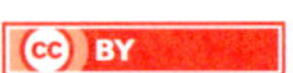

Individual chapters of this publication are distributed under the terms of the Creative Commons Attribution 3.0 Unported License which permits commercial use, distribution and reproduction of the individual chapters, provided the original author(s) and source publication are appropriately acknowledged. If so indicated, certain images may not be included under the Creative Commons license. In such cases users will need to obtain permission from the license holder to reproduce the material. More details and guidelines concerning content reuse and adaptation can be found at http://www.intechopen.com/copyright-policy.html.

Notice
Statements and opinions expressed in the chapters are these of the individual contributors and not necessarily those of the editors or publisher. No responsibility is accepted for the accuracy of information contained in the published chapters. The publisher assumes no responsibility for any damage or injury to persons or property arising out of the use of any materials, instructions, methods or ideas contained in the book.

First published in London, United Kingdom, 2020 by IntechOpen
IntechOpen is the global imprint of INTECHOPEN LIMITED, registered in England and Wales, registration number: 11086078, 7th floor, 10 Lower Thames Street, London, EC3R 6AF, United Kingdom
Printed in Croatia

British Library Cataloguing-in-Publication Data
A catalogue record for this book is available from the British Library

Additional hard and PDF copies can be obtained from orders@intechopen.com

Diseases of Pleura
Edited by Jelena Stojšić
p. cm.
Print ISBN 978-1-78985-385-8
Online ISBN 978-1-78985-386-5
eBook (PDF) ISBN 978-1-78985-467-1

For EU product safety concerns:
IN TECH d.o.o., Prolaz Marije Krucifikse Kozulić 3, 51000 Rijeka, Croatia, info@intechopen.com or visit our website at intechopen.com.

We are IntechOpen,
the world's leading publisher of
Open Access books
Built by scientists, for scientists

4,600+
Open access books available

120,000+
International authors and editors

135M+
Downloads

151
Countries delivered to

Our authors are among the
Top 1%
most cited scientists

12.2%
Contributors from top 500 universities

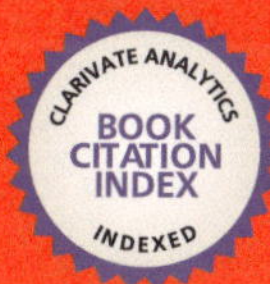

WEB OF SCIENCE™

Selection of our books indexed in the Book Citation Index
in Web of Science™ Core Collection (BKCI)

Interested in publishing with us?
Contact book.department@intechopen.com

Numbers displayed above are based on latest data collected.
For more information visit www.intechopen.com

Meet the editor

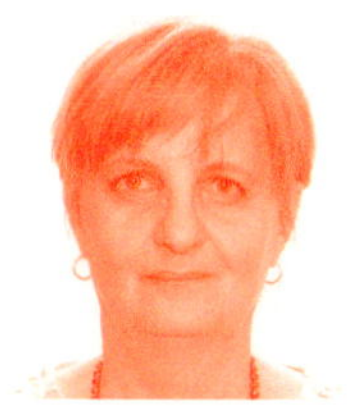

Jelena Stojšić has been a thoracic pathologist for the last 25 years. Her major interest is in the field of lung pathology, particularly lung cancer, pleural tumors, and interstitial lung diseases. The aim of her PhD thesis was recognition of the link between molecular pathways in lung cancer and transport pumps involved in the reflux of chemotherapeutics from malignant cells. In daily practice, she is involved in lung cancer pathological diagnosis based on its morphology and immunoprofile with the aim of personalizing therapy for patients. She is the author of a chapter on lung cancer for IntechOpen and the editor of book on interstitial lung disease.

Contents

Preface

Pleural diseases are usually accompanied by pulmonary or nonpulmonary (heart, kidney, thyroid, systemic) diseases. Rarely, pleural diseases are solitary lesions. Pleural effusions are frequent manifestations of pleural diseases. In this book the authors attempt to get closer to the cause of pleural effusions as well as their treatment. They also try to get closer to the complications of prolonged and untreated pleural inflammation. Some chapters describe the diagnosis and treatment of pleural tumors, both common and uncommon.

The introductory chapter describes the diagnosis and treatment of pleural tumors.

The authors of the first chapter aim to present the risk of developing asbestos related pleural diseases which may be influenced by asbestos exposure, genetic factors, interactions between different genetic factors, as well as interactions between different genetic factors and asbestos exposure. It is the purpose of the second chapter describe the effects of talc, particularly cosmetic talcum powders in the causation of diseases of the pleura. The management of bronchopleural fistula is one of the most complex challenges encountered by the thoracic surgeons and so its prevention is the best way to manage it and it is the topic of the third chapter in this book.

The last chapter as well as the intro chapter describes the diagnosis and treatment of pleural tumors, both of common and uncommon type.

I hope that this book will be used as a manual to help all physicians in everyday practice. I would like to thank all the authors who devoted their effort and time in shaping and writing their chapters. I wish all of them great success in their practice.

Jelena Stojšić, MD PhD
Head of Department of Thoracopulmonary Pathology,
Service of Pathology,
Clinical Center of Serbia,
Belgrade, Serbia

Chapter 1

Introductory Chapter: Pathology of the Pleura

Jelena Stojšić

1. Pathology of the pleura

Pleural disorders are always in the shadow of lung diseases. The discussion of these diseases has been neglected in relation to other diseases although the symptoms of pleural effusion always accompany lung as well as heart diseases.

Inflammation of the pleura may be acute or chronic, of nonspecific or specific type. Prolonged, chronic effusion causes reactive changes on mesothelial cells that can be histologically misdiagnosed as malignancy. Tuberculosis inflammation causes pleural effusion characterized by the presence of large numbers of lymphocytes and a small number of mesothelial cells. Tuberculous pleuritis is the most common form of extrapulmonary tuberculosis [1].

Malignant pleural effusions are a consequence of lung cancer spreading to visceral or parietal pleura. Pleural mesothelioma also causes effusions [2, 3].

The most accurate differential diagnosis between primary lung cancer and pleural mesothelioma is immunohistochemical diagnosis [4–7].

Pleural tumors originate from mesenchymal cells of the epithelial type and submesothelial cells of the mesenchymal type. The most common pleural mesenchymal tumor is a solitary fibrous tumor of the pleura. The biological behavior of this tumor of the pleura is predicted by the proliferation marker, protein Ki-67, and when its index is more than 4 mitoses at 2 mm^2 or >4/10 high power fields, it may be considered as a malignant alteration that creates dilemmas about the treatment [8, 9].

We will pay particular attention to reactive mesothelial cells as well as to tumors of the pleura.

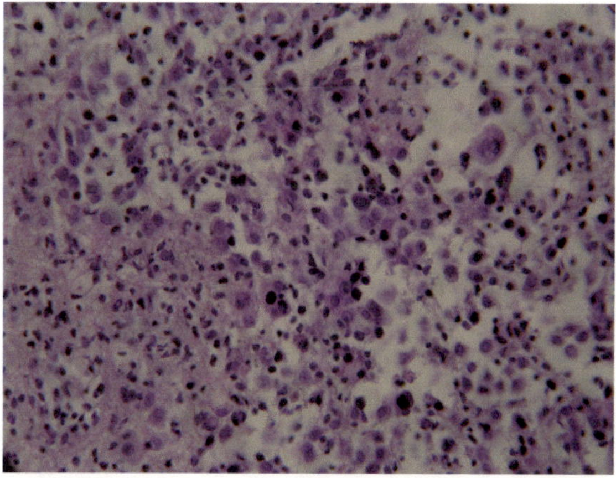

Figure 1.
Cellular pleural effusion with mass of reactive mesothelial cells.

IntechOpen

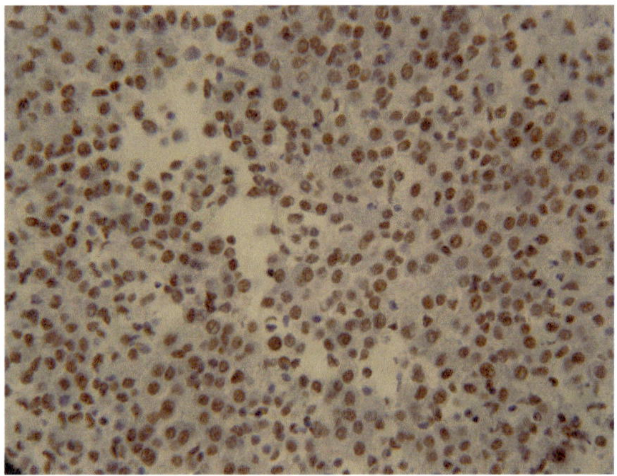

Figure 2.
Bap-1 is a protein expressed in reactive mesothelial cells.

Reactively altered mesothelial cells are difficult to distinguish morphologically from malignant mesothelial cells both on biopsy and on effusion (**Figure 1**) [8, 9]. Recently, a monoclonal antibody, bap-1, which is mainly expressed in reactive mesothelial cells has been used (**Figure 2**). It is also expressed in malignant mesothelial cells but not in malignant cells of another origin, such as lung adenocarcinoma [10].

According to the latest WHO classification of pleural tumors [8], they are divided into mesothelial tumors, mesenchymal tumors, and lymphoproliferative disorders.

2. Classification of pleural tumors

- **Mesothelial tumors**
    - Diffuse malignant mesothelioma
    - Epithelioid mesothelioma
    - Sarcomatoid mesothelioma
    - Biphasic mesothelioma
    - Desmoplastic mesothelioma
    - Localized malignant mesothelioma
    - Other tumors of mesothelial origin
    - Well-differentiated papillary mesothelioma
    - Adenomatoid tumor

- **Lymphoproliferative disorders**
    - Primary effusion lymphoma
    - Pyothorax—associated with lymphoma
- **Mesenchymal tumors**
    - Epithelioid hemangioendothelioma
    - Angiosarcoma
    - Synovial sarcoma
    - Monophasic
    - Biphasic
    - Solitary fibrous tumor
    - Calcifying tumor of pleura
    - Desmoplastic round cell tumor

We will consider the most common types, in the group of mesothelial tumors—pleural mesothelioma and in the group of mesenchymal tumors—solitary fibrous tumor.

Pleural mesothelioma is divided into the most common, monophasic, epithelioid type (**Figure 3**); sarcomatoid type (**Figure 4**); biphasic, epithelioid/sarcomatoid (**Figure 5**) and the rarest, difficult-to-diagnose, desmoplastic type (**Figure 6**). Epithelioid mesothelioma is diagnosed and differentiated from carcinoma that involve pleura with monoclonal antibodies: podoplanin (D2-40) (**Figure 7**), HBME-1 (**Figure 8**), cytokeratin 5 (**Figure 9**), calretinin (**Figure 10**), and WT-1 (**Figure 11**). By using several of these antibodies, epithelioid mesothelioma can be diagnosed with great certainty. Sarcomatoid mesothelioma can be diagnosed by using the following antibodies: cytokeratin, vimentin, HBME-1, and Fascin, but this type can be differentiated from pulmonary sarcomatoid carcinoma only by clinical findings [4–8].

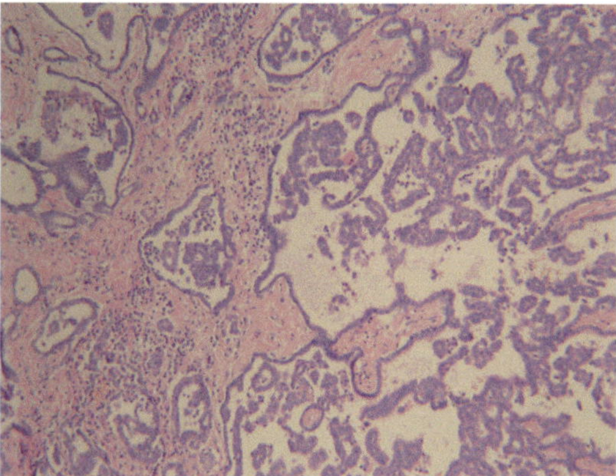

Figure 3.
The most frequent type is epithelioid malignant mesothelioma.

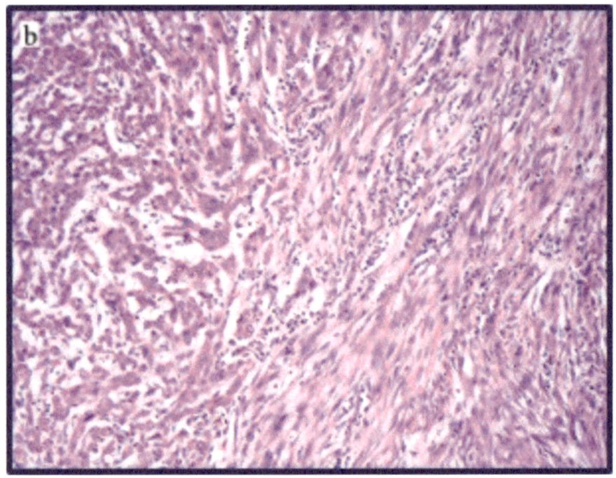

Figure 4.
Mixed, epithelioid/sarcomatoid type of malignant mesothelioma.

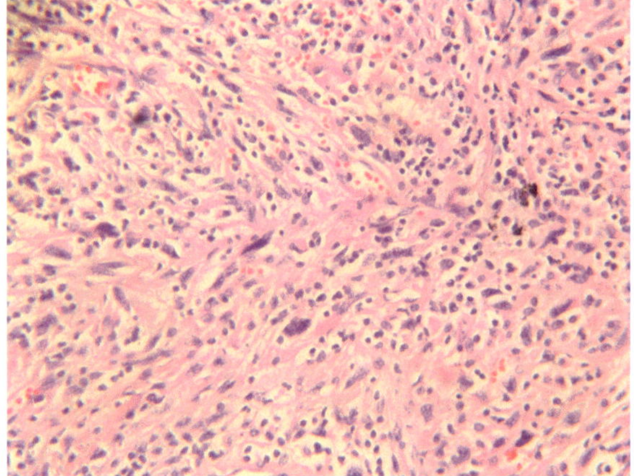

Figure 5.
Sarcomatoid type of malignant mesothelioma.

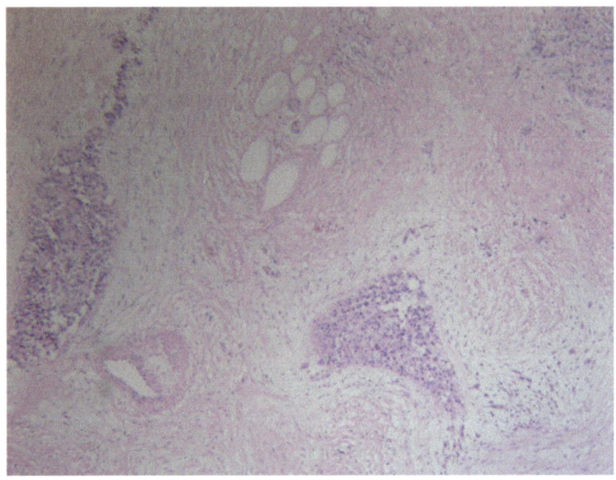

Figure 6.
Desmoplastic malignant mesothelioma is a rare type and difficult for pathological diagnosis.

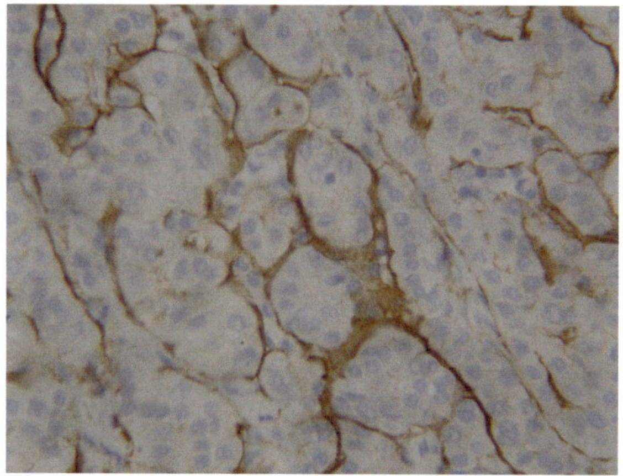

Figure 7.
Podoplanin (D2-40) is characteristic antibody for diagnosis of epithelioid type of malignant mesothelioma.

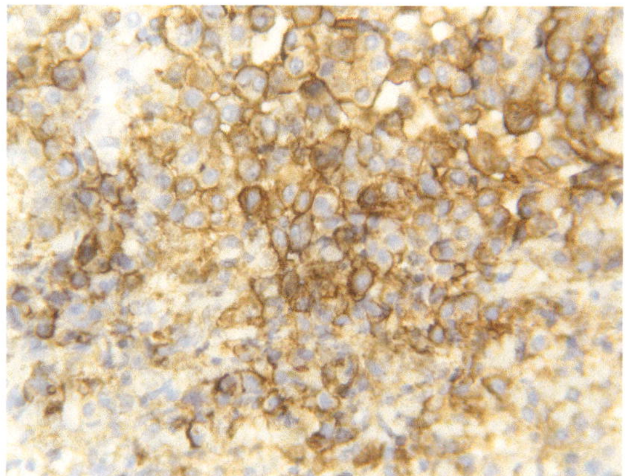

Figure 8.
HBME-1 is useful antibody for diagnosis of epithelioid type of malignant mesothelioma.

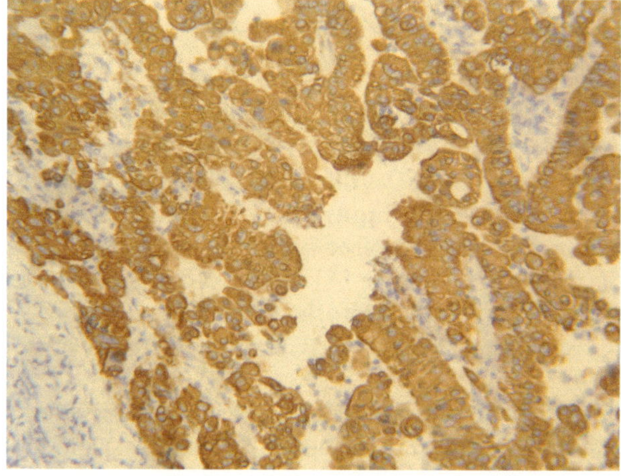

Figure 9.
Cytokeratin 5 is dominant antibody for diagnosis of epithelioid type of malignant mesothelioma.

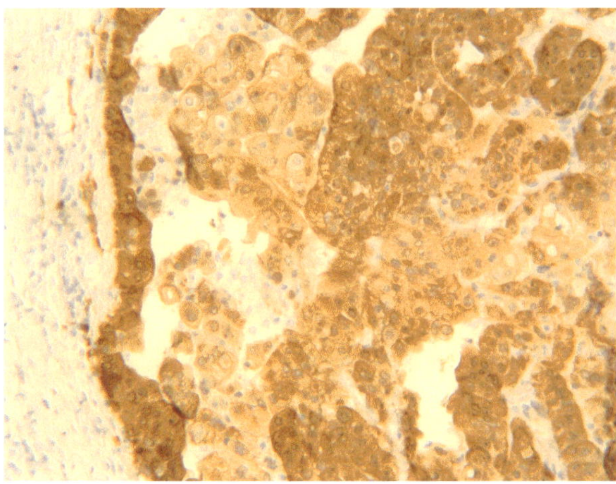

Figure 10.
Calretinin is useful for diagnosis of epithelioid type of malignant mesothelioma but could be expressed in lung adenocarcinoma.

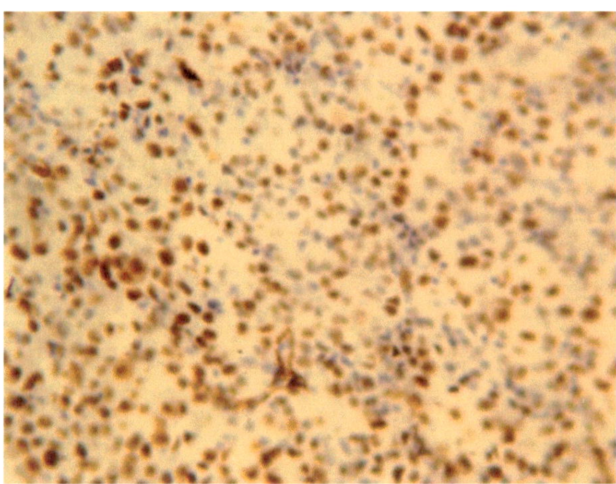

Figure 11.
WT-1 is dominant antibody for diagnosis of epithelioid type of malignant mesothelioma.

Solitary fibrous tumor is fibroblastic neoplasm, consisting of primitive connective tissue cells, which can therefore mimic morphological picture of neurofibroma or hemangiopericytoma with zones of hypercellularity (**Figure 12**) and hypocellularity (**Figure 13**). However, solitary fibrous tumor is characterized by immunophenotype of tumor cells. These cells express vimentin, CD34, bcl-2, and Stat-6 (**Figure 14**). The proliferation index of these cells is low in benign phase, less than 2 mitosis/10 HPF (**Figure 15**). If this tumor recurs and proliferation index is elevated, it is advised that tumor is treated as a sarcoma [11, 12].

Rare mesenchymal tumors are epithelioid hemangioendotheliomas which can be bilateral, both in the lungs and in the pleura. Monophasic and biphasic types of synovial sarcoma are also rare. These tumors have a specific immunophenotype, where epithelioid hemangioendothelioma (**Figures 16–18**) expresses vascular markers, while synovial sarcoma expresses (**Figures 19** and **20**) itself as synovial sarcoma of the joints but with a specific genetic mutation [13–15].

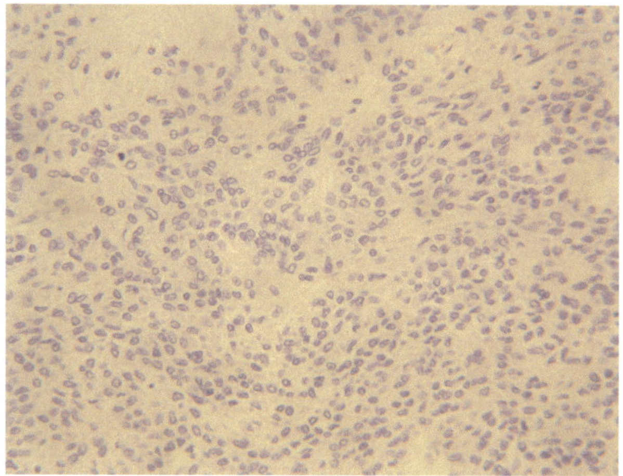

Figure 12.
Hypercellular zone of solitary fibrous tumor of pleura.

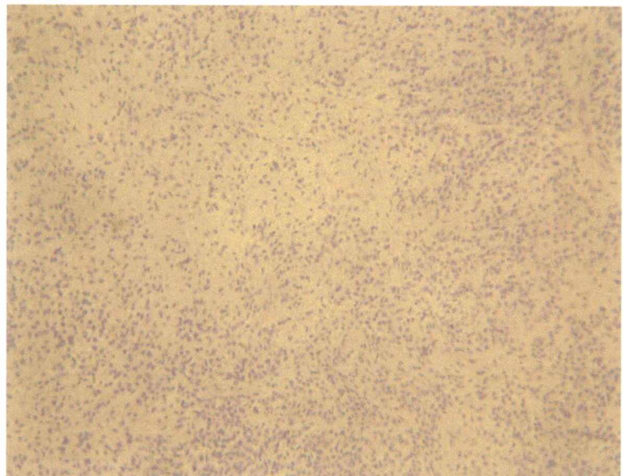

Figure 13.
Hypocellular zone of solitary fibrous tumor of pleura.

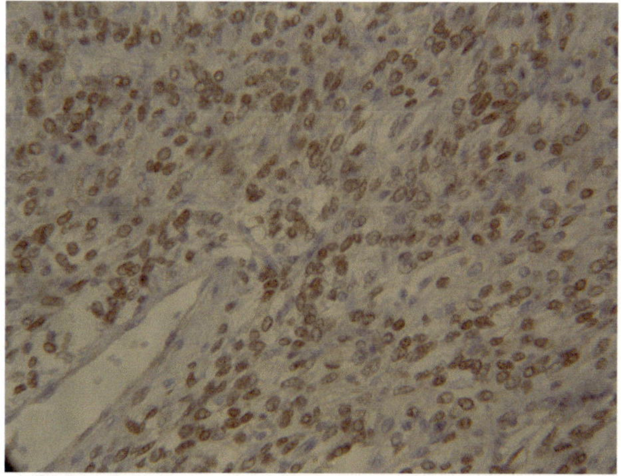

Figure 14.
Stat-6 is a characteristic antibody for diagnosis of solitary fibrous tumor of pleura.

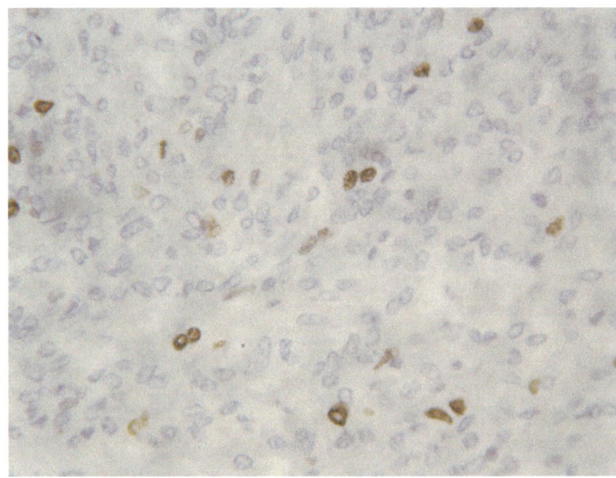

Figure 15.
High Ki-67 proliferative index (>4/10 high power fields), is a sign of malignant alteration of solitary fibrous tumor of pleura.

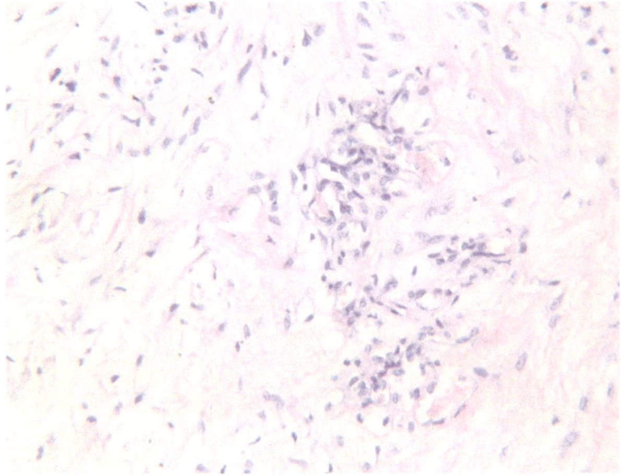

Figure 16.
Small cleft covered focally by with "signet ring cell" appearance in epithelioid hemangioendothelioma.

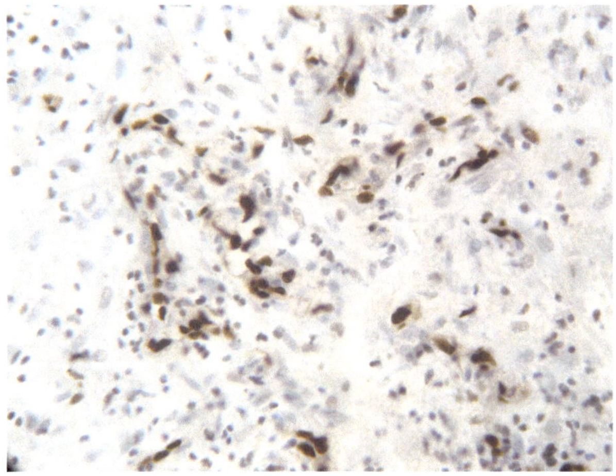

Figure 17.
Fli-1 expression in cells confirmed endothelial cells.

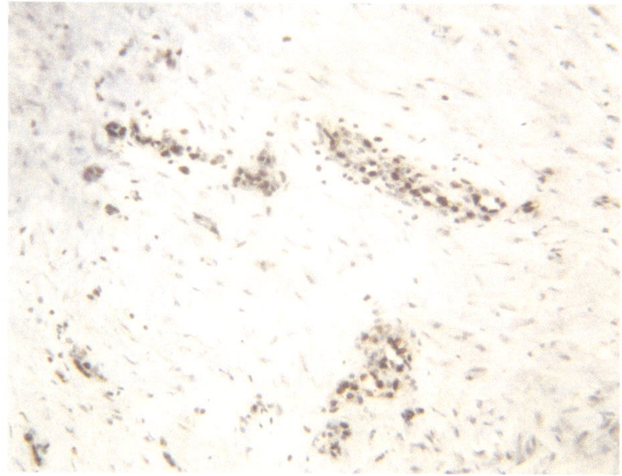

Figure 18.
ERG expression also confirmed endothelial origin of the tumor cells.

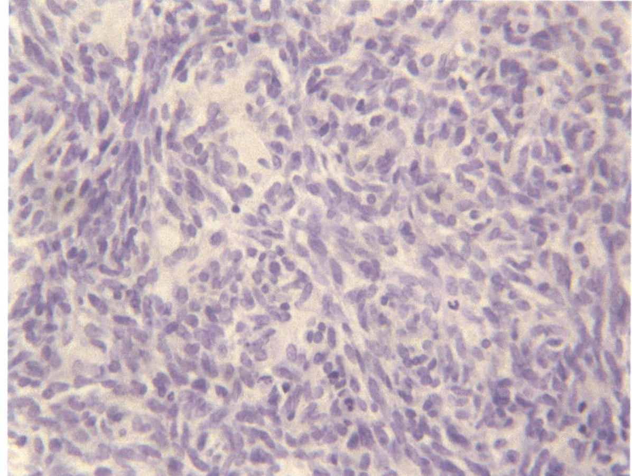

Figure 19.
Small spindle cells in sarcomatoid type of synoviosarcoma.

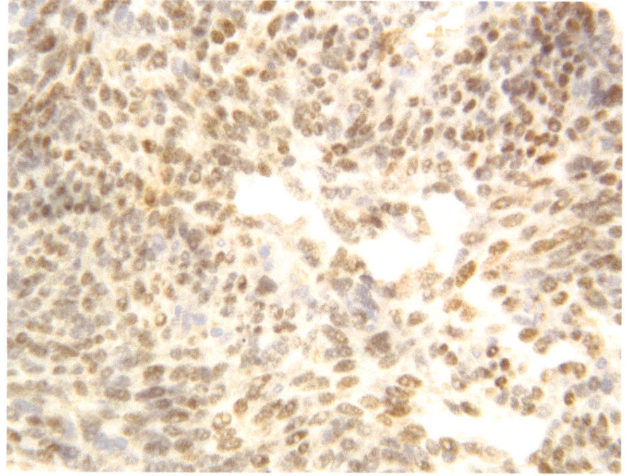

Figure 20.
Tle-1 is expressed in synoviosarcoma.

Author details

Jelena Stojšić
Service of Pathology, University Clinical Centre, Belgrade, Serbia

*Address all correspondence to: dr.jelenastoj@gmail.com

IntechOpen

© 2020 The Author(s). Licensee IntechOpen. This chapter is distributed under the terms of the Creative Commons Attribution License (http://creativecommons.org/licenses/by/3.0), which permits unrestricted use, distribution, and reproduction in any medium, provided the original work is properly cited. CC BY

References

[1] Ferreiro L, San José E, Valdés L. Tuberculous pleural effusion. Archivos de Bronconeumología. 2014;**50**(10):435-443. DOI: 10.1016/j.arbres.2013.07.006

[2] Ferreiro L, San José ME, Valdés L. Management of parapneumonic pleural effusion in adults. Archivos de Bronconeumología. 2015;**51**(12):637-646. DOI: 10.1016/j.arbres.2015.01.009

[3] Ferreiro L, Porcel JM, Diagnosis VL. Management of pleural transudates. Archivos de Bronconeumología. 2017 Nov;**53**(11):629-636. DOI: 10.1016/j.arbres.2017.04.018

[4] Husain AN, Colby TV, Ordóñez NG, Allen TC, Attanoos RL, Beasley MB, et al. Guidelines for pathologic diagnosis of malignant mesothelioma 2017 update of the consensus statement from the International Mesothelioma Interest Group. Archives of Pathology & Laboratory Medicine. 2018;**142**(1):89-108. DOI: 10.5858/arpa.2017-0124-RA

[5] Travis WD, Brambilla E, Nicholson AG, Yatabe Y, Austin JHM, Beasley MB, et al. The 2015 World Health Organization Classification of Lung Tumors: Impact of genetic, clinical and radiologic advances since the 2004 classification. Journal of Thoracic Oncology. 2015;**10**(9):1243-1260. DOI: 10.1097/JTO.0000000000000630

[6] Karpathiou G, Stefanou D, Froudarakis ME. Pleural neoplastic pathology. Respiratory Medicine. 2015;**109**(8):931-943. DOI: 10.1016/j.rmed.2015.05.014

[7] Venkatachala S, Shivakumar S, Prabhu M, Padilu R. Histomorphological and immunohistochemical analysis of pleural neoplasms. Iranian Journal of Pathology. 2018;**13**(2):196-204

[8] Travis WD, Brambila E, Burke AP, Marx A, Nicholson AG, editors. WHO Classification of Tumors of Lung, Pleura, Thymus and Heart. 4th ed. Lyon: IARC; 2015

[9] Diebold M, Soltermann A, Hottinger S, Haile SR, Bubendorf L, Komminoth P, et al. Prognostic value of MIB-1 proliferation index in solitary fibrous tumors of the pleura implemented in a new score—A multicenter study. Respiratory Research. 2017;**18**(1):210. DOI: 10.1186/s12931-017-0693-8

[10] Cigognetti M, Lonardi S, Fisogni S, Balzarini P, Pellegrini V, Tironi A, et al. BAP1 (BRCA1-associated protein 1) is a highly specific marker for differentiating mesothelioma from reactive mesothelial proliferations. Modern Pathology. 2015;**28**(8):1043-1057. DOI: 10.1038/modpathol.2015.65

[11] Vogels RJ, Vlenterie M, Versleijen-Jonkers YM, Ruijter E, Bekers EM, Verdijk MA, et al. Solitary fibrous tumor—Clinicopathologic, immunohistochemical and molecular analysis of 28 cases. Diagnostic Pathology. 2014;**9**:224. DOI: 10.1186/s13000-014-0224-6

[12] Ali SZ, Hoon V, Hoda S, Heelan R, Zakowski MF. Solitary fibrous tumor. A cytologic-histologic study with clinical, radiologic, and immunohistochemical correlations. Cancer. 1997;**81**(2):116-121

[13] Lan T, Chen H, Xiong B, Zhou T, Peng R, Chen M, et al. Primary pleuropulmonary and mediastinal synovial sarcoma: A clinicopathologic and molecular study of 26 genetically confirmed cases in the largest institution of southwest China. Diagnostic Pathology. 2016;**11**:62. DOI: 10.1186/s13000-016-0513-3

[14] Kim GH, Kim MY, Koo HJ, Song JS, Choi CM. Primary pulmonary synovial sarcoma in a tertiary referral center:

Clinical characteristics, CT, and ^{18}F-FDG PET findings, with pathologic correlations. Medicine (Baltimore). 2015;**94**(34):e1392. DOI: 10.1097/MD.0000000000001392

[15] Attanoos RL, Suvarna SK, Rhead E, Stephens M, Locke TJ, Sheppard MN, et al. Malignant vascular tumors of the pleura in “asbestos” workers and endothelial differentiation in malignant mesothelioma. Thorax. 2000;**55**(10):860-863

Chapter 2

Asbestos-Related Pleural Diseases: The Role of Gene-Environment Interactions

Vita Dolzan and Alenka Franko

Abstract

Several pleural diseases have been associated with asbestos exposure. Asbestos exposure may lead to the development of benign pleural diseases, such as pleural plaques, diffuse pleural thickening, and pleural effusion, as well as to the development of malignant mesothelioma, a highly aggressive tumour of the pleura. Asbestos exposure related to pleural diseases may be occupational or environmental. Although the causal relationship between asbestos-related pleural diseases and asbestos exposure has been well confirmed, the role of genetic factors in the development of these diseases needs to be further investigated and elucidated. The results of the studies performed so far indicate that in addition to asbestos exposure, genetic factors as well as the interactions between genetic factors and asbestos exposure may have an important impact on the risk of asbestos-related pleural diseases, especially malignant mesothelioma. This chapter aims to present how the risk of developing asbestos-related pleural diseases may be influenced by asbestos exposure, genetic factors, interactions between different genetic factors, as well as interactions between different genetic factors and asbestos exposure.

Keywords: pleural plaques, malignant mesothelioma, asbestos exposure, genetic factors

1. Introduction

Asbestos-related diseases still represent an important health problem and a huge economic burden for the society all over the world. Asbestos exposure has been associated with the development of asbestosis, pleural plaques, diffuse pleural thickening and pleural effusion, lung cancer, malignant mesothelioma of pleura and peritoneum, and several other types of cancers, like laryngeal cancer, ovarian cancer, as well as cancers of the buccal mucosa, pharynx, gastrointestinal tract, and kidney [1–13].

Asbestos-related diseases, including those of the pleura, are known to be among the most investigated occupational diseases [8–14].

2. Asbestos-related pleural diseases

Development of several pleural diseases has been associated with occupational or environmental asbestos exposure. Among them are pleural plaques, diffuse pleural thickening, pleural effusion, and malignant mesothelioma of the pleura [1–7].

2.1 Pleural plaques

Pleural plaques are benign (nonmalignant) pleural abnormalities and among the most common asbestos-related diseases [15–17].

Pleural plaques have been defined as circumscribed, quadrangular, irregular pleural elevations with clearly demarcated edges that are often bilateral and rarely symmetrical. They may enlarge and become calcified over time. Pleural plaques commonly develop in the lower two thirds of the thorax and mostly on the outer two thirds of diaphragm. They rarely occur within less than 20 years from the first exposure to asbestos [3, 5, 15–19].

Pleural plaques are mostly asymptomatic and may cause a slight impairment of lung function when they grow in size [20].

Small pleural plaques are often difficult to discern, and standard chest radiographs are generally suboptimal for the visualisation of pleura, particularly in obese patients [3]. High-resolution CT (HRCT) scans are far superior to any other method for imaging pleural plaques as well as the diffuse pleural thickening [3, 21].

Pleural plaques have been referred predominately as a marker of asbestos exposure [2, 5, 22, 23] rather than an independent risk factor for malignant mesothelioma and lung cancer [2, 5, 24]. However, according to some authors, pleural plaques may also indicate an increased risk of asbestosis and asbestos-related cancers [18, 19]. Many studies have investigated the relationship between pleural plaques and lung cancer as well as between pleural plaques and malignant mesothelioma; however, the results of these studies are not consistent [5, 24].

Regarding the relation between pleural plaques and malignant mesothelioma, Hillerdal et al. reported that pleural plaques on the chest roentgenogram indicate an increased risk for mesothelioma [25]. In their study Karjalainen et al. presented more than five times higher risk of malignant mesothelioma in asbestos-exposed men with benign pleural disease [26]. A statistically significant association between pleural plaques and malignant mesothelioma (unadjusted), and after adjustment for the time since the first exposure and the cumulative exposure index to asbestos, was observed also in the study of Pairon et al. Based on these results, Pairon et al. concluded that the presence of pleural plaques may be an independent risk factor for pleural mesothelioma [27]. On the other hand, Reid et al. reported no increased risk of pleural malignant mesothelioma in subjects with pleural thickening after adjustment for the time since the first exposure (log years), cumulative exposure (log f/ml-years), and age at the start of the programme; however, there was an increased risk of peritoneal mesothelioma [28].

Considering lung cancer, Fletcher reported two times higher risk of developing this malignoma in shipyard workers with pleural plaques compared to those without plaques [29]. Hillerdal et al. suggested that the risk for bronchial carcinoma may be increased in subjects with pleural plaques observed on the chest roentgenogram [25]. A slightly elevated risk of lung cancer was found in the asbestos-exposed men with benign pleural disease also in the study of Karjalainen et al. [26]. In the study of Cullen et al., asbestos-exposed smokers with pleural plaques or other asbestos-related pleural changes had a 44% higher risk of lung cancer than the unexposed heavy smokers [30]. Lung cancer mortality was significantly associated with pleural plaques when unadjusted and also after adjustment for smoking and asbestos cumulative exposure index in the follow-up study of Pairon et al. They concluded that pleural plaques may be an independent risk factor for lung cancer death in asbestos-exposed workers and could be used as an additional criterion in the definition of high-risk populations eligible for CT screening [27]. On the contrary, the study of Partanen et al. showed no increased risk of lung cancer in subjects with pleural plaques [31].

Nevertheless, although pleural plaques may be the endpoint and the development of pleural plaques may be an entirely independent process from the development of malignant mesothelioma and lung cancer, it is likely there is a link between pleural plaques and the aforementioned malignant diseases [5].

2.2 Diffuse pleural thickening

Diffuse pleural thickening that affects visceral pleural surface is not sharply demarcated and is often associated with fibrous strands extending into the parenchyma. There are frequent adhesions between the visceral and parietal pleurae, leading to obliteration of the pleural space. It can be extensive and cover the whole lobe or even the whole lung. The thickness ranges from less than 1 mm up to 1 cm or more. Diffuse pleural thickening is a less frequent manifestation of asbestos exposure than pleural plaques [15, 32–34].

Diffuse pleural thickening may lead to significant respiratory disability. In subjects with diffuse pleural thickening, forced vital capacity and single breath diffusing capacity are considered to be lower in comparison to subjects without this disorder [35–37].

From the diagnostic point of view, a chest radiograph is used as a standard method for detecting diffuse pleural thickenings; however, also in this case, HRCT scans are far superior to any other method [20, 37, 38].

Similar to pleural plaques, the diffuse pleural thickenings may be also associated with malignant diseases [20].

2.3 Pleural effusion

Asbestos-related changes of pleura include also benign asbestos pleural effusion, which is a nonmalignant pleural disease [39]. It has been first described in 1964, and it is also known as asbestos pleurisy [39, 40].

Diagnostic criteria for asbestos pleural effusion include previous asbestos exposure, determination of pleural effusion by chest radiograph, HRCT or thoracocentesis, and the absence of other causes of effusion [39]. In the vast majority of undiagnosed unilateral pleural effusions, the fluid is sent for cytological analysis. However, there still remains an uncertainty about the sensitivity to diagnose malignant pleural effusion. It is important to know that in patients presenting with clinical suspicion of malignant mesothelioma, cytological sensitivity is low [41].

Nevertheless, unexplained pleural effusion and pleural pain in subjects exposed to asbestos should always raise the suspicion of pleural malignant mesothelioma [42]. Sneddon et al. reported that more than 70% of patients with malignant mesothelioma develop pleural effusions, which contain tumour cells, representing a readily accessible source of malignant cells for genetic analysis [43].

2.4 Malignant mesothelioma

Malignant mesothelioma is a rare but highly aggressive and fatal cancer of serosal surfaces with poor prognosis, related to occupational and/or environmental (nonoccupational) asbestos exposure. It arises most commonly from mesothelium of the pleural surface. Rarely, it may occur also in other serosal membranes of the human body that are also coated with mesothelium, such as peritoneum, pericardium, and tunica vaginalis [44–46].

The major cause and carcinogen for the development of malignant mesothelioma is asbestos. In the study of McDonald et al., asbestos exposure was proved in almost 80% of patients with malignant mesothelioma [47]. Additionally in the study of Franko et al., asbestos exposure was confirmed in 86% of patients with malignant mesothelioma, but it could not be confirmed with certainty in the remainder of the patients [48].

The latency period between the first exposure to asbestos and the development of malignant mesothelioma is long and can range from 15 to 60 years or even more [48–50].

Considering clinical features, in the vast majority of patients, the onset of symptoms is insidious and nonspecific, with chest pain and breathlessness being the most common features [51]. These symptoms are usually mild at the onset of the disease and are often attributed to other causes, which delays the diagnosis. The chest pain is often described as a sensation of heaviness or coldness in one side of chest or abdomen and can be caused by the effusion or the tumour [51–53]. The referral of this unspecified pain to the upper abdomen or shoulders, probably as a result of involvement of the diaphragmatic pleura, may lead to the inappropriate investigation and consequently delays the diagnosis. Breathlessness may be manifested as the new onset of dyspnoea or the deterioration of the symptoms of other respiratory diseases such as chronic obstructive pulmonary disease. The latter results in further diagnostic delays [51, 54]. Another feature during the course of this cancer is a dry cough, which is rarely troublesome in the early stages and is seen in about 10% of patients [51, 55]. Other relatively common features are weight loss, fatigue, anorexia, sweats, malaise, lassitude, and intermittent low-grade fever [51, 56]. Malignant mesothelioma is occasionally found incidentally during radiological investigation of some other health problems. Another rather rare presentation of this malignoma is pneumothorax [51].

The most common form of spread of malignant mesothelioma in addition to the worsening of the presenting symptoms is dysphagia due to esophageal compression, sympathetic nerve involvement of the arm, neurological syndromes such as Horners's syndrome, recurrent laryngeal nerve palsy, paraplegia as a result of spinal canal invasion, severe pain in the chest wall as a consequence of tumour invasion and nerve root involvement, malignant pericardial invasion and effusion, obstruction of superior venal cava, and occurrence of intermittent hypoglycemia [51, 53].

A rapid and accurate diagnosis of malignant mesothelioma is very important for therapeutic reasons [44]. Pleural pain and unexplained pleural effusion in subjects exposed to asbestos should raise the suspicion of pleural malignant mesothelioma. Chest radiography, which is a simple and easily available tool, is usually the first investigation performed. The typical findings are pleural effusion, occasionally nodular pleural thickening, irregular fissural thickening, or a localised mass lesion [57]. Important imaging modality is HRCT scanning, which at the diagnosis often shows pleural effusion at disease site, pleural thickening, as well as involvement of the interlobar fissure and invasion of the chest wall. As for MRI, it has superior soft tissue contrast over CT. Diffusion-weighted MRI is considered to be a promising strategy for evaluating tumour extension and response to treatment [57]. Another method is PET-CT, which combines HRCT scanning with injection of 18-fluorodeoxy-glucose; however, also this scan has several limitations as it cannot differentiate between pleural malignant mesothelioma and metastatic pleural malignancy [57].

Invasive procedures are needed for prompt and accurate diagnosis of pleural malignant mesothelioma. Cytological samples are obtained by thoracentesis and biological tissue by ultrasound-/or radiological-guided biopsy or thoracoscopy [57]. Based on histopathology, malignant mesotheliomas can be classified into epithelioid, biphasic, and sarcomatoid subtypes [45]. However, this aggressive cancer remains difficult to diagnose in the early phases of the disease. Therefore, potential serum markers that could facilitate an early diagnosis and help to evaluate response to treatment have been extensively investigated. Among them are mesothelin [48, 58–60], fibulin-3

[61, 62], osteopontin [51], survivin [63], and others. However, the results of the studies on tumour markers are not consistent; therefore further research is needed.

Pleural malignant mesothelioma is treated by surgery, also used in combination with chemotherapy and/or radiotherapy, which attempts to eradicate the malignant tissue and is an essential option to help the patient to reduce the pain and control pleural effusions [46, 53]. Radiotherapy is relatively common treatment for pleural malignant mesothelioma. Although several studies have indicated that radiotherapy is unable to cure this cancer, it has been shown that radiotherapy administrated pre- or postoperatively alone or in combination with other treatments, is useful to limit tumour spreading, controls pain, and improves the 2-year rate of overall survival from 20 to 34% [46, 64]. However, the systemic cytotoxic chemotherapy remains one of the few therapeutic options that has been shown to improve survival in patients with malignant pleural mesothelioma even in advance stage, when patients are not candidates for aggressive surgery [46, 65]. The most commonly used is the combination of pemetrexed with cisplatin and gemcitabine with cisplatin or another platinum compound. It was reported that the combination of cisplatin and pemetrexed gave a 3-month survival benefit over cisplatin alone, improving median survival from 9.3 to 12.1 months [66]. Comparable results were obtained for gemcitabine/cisplatin doublet [67–70]. Furthermore, the introduction of chemotherapy, in particular treatment with low-dose gemcitabine in prolonged infusion and cisplatin significantly improved survival of Slovenian malignant mesothelioma patients with median overall survival being increased from 5.6 to 14.5 months [68].

3. Asbestos exposure and pleural diseases

Asbestos is a commercial collective name for a group of naturally occurring fibrous hydrated silicates that share similar physical and chemical properties [13, 71–75]. According to their fibre morphology, asbestos fibres have been sub-classified into two main groups, serpentine and amphibole. Serpentine asbestos includes chrysotile, which is also known as white asbestos. The vast category of amphiboles includes commercial asbestos crocidolite (also named blue asbestos), amosite (also called brown asbestos), anthophyllite, as well as the noncommercial types of asbestos like actinolite and tremolite asbestos [13, 75–80].

These fibres have been greatly valued for their tensile strength, thermal resistance, durability, and flexibility. However, on the other hand, asbestos fibres are known to cause inflammation, fibrotic changes in the lung, and malignant diseases [71, 72, 75].

Asbestos exposure related to asbestos-related pleural diseases, as well as to other asbestos-related diseases, may be occupational or/and environmental.

Workers may be occupationally exposed to asbestos in many working sectors, including disposal of asbestos waste and materials; construction; asbestos-cement industry; brickworks; asphalt mixing; machine and insulation products industry; production of clutches and brakes; bus, lorry, railway carriage, car, and airplane repair; ship repair and building; textile industry; asbestos mining, production and milling of asbestos fibres; textile industry; and other sectors [73–75, 77, 81–83].

Environmental (nonoccupational) exposure to asbestos (in the neighbourhood or household) occurs in the vicinity of the factories and other working sectors where asbestos is used. In these areas inhabitants are exposed to asbestos with polluted air, water, and food. Nonoccupational exposure to asbestos may also occur due to the use and improper removal of asbestos-cement roofing, asbestos insulation, and other products containing asbestos. Asbestos fibres can be found in water that runs on asbestos-cement tubes, especially if they do not have lining or if they are damaged. Family members of workers who work with asbestos and bring asbestos home with clothes, shoes, and hair can also be exposed to asbestos [13, 81–83].

Although the causal relationship between asbestos-related pleural diseases and asbestos exposure has been well confirmed, the role of genetic factors in the development of these diseases needs to be further investigated and elucidated.

3.1 Molecular mechanisms linking asbestos exposure and pleural diseases

Recent studies have led to a better understanding of molecular mechanisms underlying the pathogenesis of asbestos-related diseases, including malignant mesothelioma. Although it has been shown that asbestos fibres deposited in lungs and translocated to pleura may have direct genotoxic effects on epithelial and mesothelial cells, the main molecular mechanism linking asbestos exposure with fibroplasia and neoplasia is related to the generation of reactive oxygen and nitric species thus leading to oxidative stress and inflammation [84].

Reactive oxygen species (ROS) such as hydrogen peroxide (H_2O_2), superoxide anion ($O_2^{\,-}$), hydroxyl radical (OH•), and reactive nitrogen species (RNS) can be generated directly by the asbestos fibres as they contain redox-active iron (Fe^{2+}, Fe^{3+}) that may catalyse the formation of hydroxyl radical through Fenton reaction [85]. Secondly, ROS may be generated also indirectly by inflammatory cells such as macrophages during the frustrated phagocytosis of asbestos fibres. This process also leads to the release of proinflammatory cytokines that further potentiate the asbestos-related inflammatory response [86].

Another recently described molecular mechanism by which asbestos may contribute to inflammation is the activation of the so-called pattern recognition receptors that sense pathogen-associated or damage-associated molecular patterns (PAMPs or DAMPs, respectively) and trigger cellular responses. One class of these receptors, the nucleotide binding and oligomerization domain (NOD)-like receptors (NLRs), has been shown to be directly activated by asbestos fibres [87]. NLRP3 inflammasomes may be activated also indirectly by the released ROS and proinflammatory cytokines such as high-mobility group box 1 protein (HMGB1) [88]. Activation of NLR triggers assembly and activation of a multiprotein complex composed of the NLRP3 scaffold protein, CARD containing adaptor protein, and caspase-1. The subsequent cleavage and activation of caspase-1 lead to the downstream cleavage of pro-interleukin-1β (pro-IL-1β) and release of mature proinflammatory cytokine IL-1β that triggers the early inflammatory response following asbestos exposure [89]. IL-1β release then leads to activation and enhanced expression of other cytokines, among them tumour necrosis factor (TNF) and transforming growth factor beta-1 (TGFB1) [90, 91]. Furthermore, TGFB1 may downregulate collagen degradation through matrix metalloproteinases (MMPs) and their inhibitors (TIMPs). Several MMPs and TIMPs play an essential role in tissue repair and remodelling. Among them, MMP1, MMP9, MMP12, and TIMP2 have been proposed to contribute to the development of pulmonary fibrosis [92].

Asbestos fibres and ROS may also activate other receptors and signalling pathways such as epidermal growth factor receptor (EGFR) and the downstream protein kinases AKT and ERK, leading to the activation of c-Fos and c-Jun proto-oncogenes and dysregulation of mitogenic signalling, promoting fibrosis and malignant transformation [93]. Because of the long-term persistence of asbestos fibres, the inflammation becomes chronic and is accompanied by gradual progression from mesothelial hyperplasia to mesothelioma after a latency period of several decades. In vitro and in vivo evidence implicate oxidative stress, chronic inflammation, genetic and epigenetic alterations, as well as direct cellular toxicity and genotoxicity as the main mechanisms in the asbestos-related development of fibrosis and in malignant mesothelial cell transformation [94].

Numerous chromosomal abnormalities and genetic and epigenetic alterations were identified in human mesothelioma tissues in asbestos-exposed workers [94]. Asbestos-induced mutagenicity is also mediated through direct or indirect pathways. Asbestos fibres may induce mutagenicity and genotoxicity directly through physical interaction with the mitotic machinery of dividing cells after being phagocytized by the target cells. Longer asbestos fibres in particular, may cause DNA double-strand breaks or interact with the mitotic spindle thus leading to aneuploidy [94]. The indirect genotoxic and mutagenic effects occur due to asbestos-generated ROS and RNS that may produce a variety of DNA and chromosomal damages, such as 8-hydroxydeoxyguanosine (8-OHdG), DNA single-strand breaks, and chromosome fragmentation. Other frequently observed genomic alteration includes homozygous deletion or change of methylation pattern of tumour suppressor and p16INK4a and p14ARF at the 9p21 locus in humans. p16INK4a/p14ARF homozygous deletion has been reported to occur at a frequency of 50–70% of MM tissues and primary MM cells, whereas in stable MM cell lines, the frequency is as high as 90%. The loss of p16INK4a/p14ARF leads to the inactivation of another two important tumour suppressors, pRB and p53. The loss of neurofibromatosis type 2 (NF2) gene leads to the deficiency of its product Merlin and the consequent loss of inhibition of Merlin's downstream target YAP, a proto-oncogene and transcriptional coactivator that promotes cell proliferation. Copy number amplification of proto-oncogenes such as JUN, MYC, and YAP was also reported [94].

Homozygous deletion of another tumour suppressor gene, BAP1, was recently reported in familial malignant mesothelioma. BAP1 is part of a multiprotein complex that is involved in DNA damage response and regulation of gene transcription [95].

3.2 The role of genetic factors in the development of asbestos-related pleural diseases

Recent studies have shown that in addition to asbestos exposure, genetic factors may have an important role in the occurrence, progression, and response to treatment of asbestos-related diseases. Most studies have focused on genetic variability, in particular genetic polymorphisms in genes involved in the pathways related to molecular mechanisms linking asbestos exposure and pleural diseases as potential candidate genes that may influence individual susceptibility to asbestos-associated disorders. Most of the studies focused on asbestosis and malignant mesothelioma as the most common respective nonmalignant and malignant diseases related to asbestos exposure, while only a small number of studies included patients with pleural thickening and pleural plaques. This chapter is leaving asbestosis-related studies aside, as they are related to interstitial and not pleural lung disease.

3.2.1 Genetic variability in antioxidative defence genes

The defence mechanism against ROS is complex and involves several enzymes. Superoxide dismutases (SODs), catalase (CAT), and glutathione peroxidases (GPX) constitute the first line of the antioxidant enzyme defence system against ROS, while glutathione S-transferases (GSTs) play an important role in the detoxification of cytotoxic secondary metabolites of ROS. The major GST enzyme in the human lung is GSTP1, which belongs to the Pi class. Two other important polymorphic GSTs are GSTM1 (Mu class) and GSTT1 (Theta class) [96]. Another Phase 2 enzyme studied in asbestos-related diseases is *N*-acetyltransferase 2 (NAT2), involved in the metabolism of various xenobiotics including the aromatic and heterocyclic amines present in tobacco smoke and the diet [97]. The genes coding for all these enzymes are known to be polymorphic. Some of these polymorphisms alter gene expression or enzymatic activity and may modify the ability for the elimination of ROS or their products [98–100].

Manganese SOD (SOD2) was found to be highly expressed in malignant mesothelioma; however, *SOD2* rs1799725 (Val16Ala) polymorphism was not found to be associated with either malignant or nonmalignant asbestos-related diseases in a group of 124 Finnish asbestos insulators, among which 20 workers developed malignant mesothelioma, 41 had nonmalignant pulmonary disorders such as asbestosis and/or pleural plaques, while 63 had no pulmonary disorders [98]. On the other hand, homozygotes for *SOD2* 16Ala/Ala genotype were found to have a threefold increased risk for malignant mesothelioma when genotype distributions were compared among 90 Italian patients with malignant mesothelioma and 395 controls [100]. In this cohort, increased risk for malignant mesothelioma was also observed in carriers of homozygous *GSTM1* deletion (*GSTM1* null genotype), while no association was observed for polymorphisms in other *GST* genes [100].

Kukkonen et al. [101] investigated nine polymorphisms in six genes (*EPHX1*, *GSTM1*, *GSTM3*, *GSTP1*, *GSTT1*, and *NAT2*) related to metabolism of oxidative species in a cohort of 1008 Finnish asbestos-exposed workers. Only a trend of association was observed between *GSTM1* null genotype and the extent of pleural plaques as well as between *GSTP1* Ile105Val polymorphism and the calcification of pleural plaques. However, when pleural plaques were stratified according to the severity of radiological changes, *GSTT1* null genotype was significantly associated with the greatest thickness of the pleural plaques [101].

No association was also found between *SOD2* and *CAT* polymorphisms and the malignant mesothelioma risk in a study that included 159 Slovenian malignant mesothelioma patients and 122 controls. All the controls were occupationally exposed to asbestos in the asbestos-cement manufacturing plant but did not develop any disease associated with asbestos exposure [102]. However, this study reported an association between NAD(P)H quinone dehydrogenase 1 (*NQO1*) rs1800566 (p.Pro187Ser) SNP and malignant mesothelioma risk. NQO1 catalyses the reduction of quinones to hydroquinones, thus preventing the formation of free radicals. The carriers of at least one polymorphic *NQO1* allele (CT and TT genotypes) had an increased risk of malignant mesothelioma compared to carriers of homozygous wild-type CC genotype [102].

In a Finnish cohort, an association was reported between the *NAT2* slow-acetylator genotype and increased risk for both malignant (mesothelioma) and nonmalignant (asbestosis and pleural plaques) pulmonary disorders among asbestos-exposed workers [103, 104]. On the contrary, the *NAT2* slow-acetylator genotypes were associated with decreased risk of mesothelioma in the Italian study population [105]. Conflicting results were reported also regarding the impact of microsomal epoxide hydrolase (EPHX1), a metabolising enzyme that plays a dual role in the activation and detoxification of exogenous chemicals, such as epoxides and PAHs [106]. *EPHX1* low-activity genotypes were positively associated with malignant mesothelioma in the Italian study population, while in the Finnish study population, the association was negative [105].

3.2.2 Genetic variability in NLRP3 inflammasome

Two polymorphic genes leading to enhanced innate immune response and increased production of inflammatory cytokines were investigated in asbestos-related pleural diseases. *NLRP3* rs35829419 (p.Gln705Lys; C > A) is a gain-of-function polymorphism that leads to increased NLRP3 activation after stimulation.

On the other hand, *CARD8* rs2043211 (p.Cys10Ter, A > T) is a loss of function SNP that results in nonfunctional protein so that the CARD-8 inhibition of caspase-1 is lost. Therefore, both SNPs are associated with proinflammatory phenotype [107, 108]. Both SNPs were analysed in a large Finnish study that investigated 16 polymorphisms from nine genes (NLRP3, CARD8, TNF, TGFB1, GC, MMP1, MMP9, MMP12, and TIMP2) involved in innate immunity and intracellular matrix remodelling in 951 Finnish asbestos-exposed workers. Among the two investigated *NLRP3* SNPs, only rs35829419 was associated with interstitial lung fibrosis but showed no association with fibrotic changes of pleura. Among the three investigated *CARD8* SNPs, rs2043211 (p.Cys10Ter, A > T) was associated with the greatest thickness of pleural plaques [107].

3.2.3 Genetic variability in signalling and inflammatory pathways

Asbestos-related activation of inflammation also leads to increased TNF and TGFB1 production. *TNF* promoter polymorphism rs1800629 (−308G > A) was reported to lead to higher constitutive and inducible transcriptional TNFa levels [109]. Genotype and allele frequencies of TNF promoter polymorphism rs1800629 (−308G > A) were associated with radiographic pleural changes among German workers occupationally exposed to asbestos. Compared with the healthy nonexposed control group, carriers of at least one polymorphic TNF −308 A allele had at higher risk for hyaline pleural plaques, while no association was observed for calcified pleural plaques [91].

TGFB1 is a multifunctional cytokine that regulates the proliferation and differentiation of cells [110] and was reported to promote the pathogenesis of lung fibrosis and act as a tumour suppressor in normal cells. Two *TGFB1* polymorphisms in codons 10 (Leu10Pro) and 25 (Arg25Pro) affecting TGFB1 protein production were associated with a higher risk for fibrotic lung diseases but a lower risk for lung cancer in a German cohort that included 591 patients with pulmonary fibrosis, 147 patients with bronchial carcinoma, and 83 healthy control subjects [90].

Kukkonen et al. investigated common polymorphisms in *TNF* and *TGFB1* genes; however, only *TGFB1* showed associations with visceral pleural fibrosis among 951 Finnish Caucasian asbestos-exposed workers. In stratified analysis carriers of at least one *TGFB1* rs2241718 variant allele were protected against visceral pleural fibrosis. On the other hand, *TGFB1* haplotype analysis showed an association with pleural plaque calcification. In particular, *TGFB1* rs1800469-rs1800470 GC and AT haplotypes conferred increased risks for pleural plaque calcification when compared with the most common haplotype, GT [107].

3.2.4 Genes involved in matrix remodelling

In the above-mentioned study, Kukkonen et al. also investigated common polymorphisms of several metalloproteinases and their inhibitors (*MMP*1 rs1799750, *MMP9* rs3918242, *MMP12* rs652438, and *TIMP2* rs2277698) involved in matrix remodelling. The study reported an association between the *TIMP2* rs2277698 SNP and pleural thickenings, and the variant allele was found to predispose to a high degree of pleural plaque calcification [107].

Strbac et al. investigated 10 different SNPs in three *MMP* genes (*MMP2*, *MMP9*, and *MMP14*) in a group of 236 Slovenian patients with malignant mesothelioma and 161 healthy blood donors as the control group. The study reported a decreased risk for malignant mesothelioma in carriers of at least one polymorphic *MMP2* rs243865 allele, and this association was even more pronounced in patients with known asbestos exposure. None of the other tested polymorphisms showed association with the risk of malignant pleural mesothelioma [111]. Furthermore, a study including 199 Slovenian malignant mesothelioma patients suggested that *MMP* polymorphisms may have a role as prognostic biomarkers in malignant mesothelioma, as carriers of polymorphic *MMP9* rs2250889 allele had shorter time to progression and shorter overall survival compared to noncarriers. In contrast, carriers of at least one polymorphic *MMP9* rs20544 allele had longer time to progression and longer OS (overall survival than noncarriers [112].

3.2.5 Genes involved in DNA repair mechanisms

It has been suggested that genetic variability of proteins involved in DNA repair mechanisms may affect the risk of malignant mesothelioma. Based on the mechanisms of either oxidative stress related or direct DNA damage discussed above, polymorphic genes in DNA repair pathways such as base excision repair (BER), nucleotide excision repair (NER), as well as homologous recombination may play a role in susceptibility to asbestos-related malignant diseases [93]. However, so far only a few studies investigated the influence of the genetic variability of proteins involved in DNA repair mechanisms on the development of malignant mesothelioma. In particular, polymorphisms in genes coding for excision repair cross-complementing group 1 protein (ERCC1) involved in NER and X-ray repair cross-complementing protein 1 (XRCC1) involved in BER were most frequently investigated in asbestos-related malignant diseases [113, 114].

Dianzani et al. investigated seven SNPs in four DNA repair genes (*XRCC1, XRCC3, XPD,* and *OGG1*) in a population-based case-control study that included 81 patients and 110 age and sex-matched controls from Casale Monferrato, an Italian town known for high levels of asbestos pollution. Two of the investigated polymorphisms were significantly associated with increased malignant mesothelioma risk in both homozygous and heterozygous carriers when compared to noncarriers: *XRCC1* rs25487 (399Q) and *XRCC3* rs861539 (241T). Homozygous and heterozygous carriers of *OGG1* rs1052133 −326C allele were also at increased risk for malignant mesothelioma; but this association did not reach statistical significance. Also, the association with malignant mesothelioma risk was not significant when *XRCC1* and *XRCC3* haplotypes were considered [113].

A follow-up study included 220 malignant mesothelioma patients and 296 controls from two Italian towns, Casale and Turin, and investigated 35 SNPs in 15 genes possibly related to asbestos carcinogenicity. Among them, 14 SNPs in 10 genes involved in DNA repair were studied; however, only three SNPs were found to be associated with malignant mesothelioma. When only asbestos-exposed patients were considered in the analysis, the risk for malignant mesothelioma was found to increase with the number of *XRCC1* rs25487 (399Q) polymorphic alleles and *XRCC1* −77T alleles. Increased risk for malignant mesothelioma was also observed in *XRCC1* haplotype analysis. *ERCC1* rs11615 (N118N) polymorphism was also found to be associated with increased malignant mesothelioma risk in the dominant genetic model, both in the entire study group and when considering only asbestos-exposed patients [114].

Betti et al. also investigated one functional SNP in *hOGG* (rs1052133 p.Ser326Cys) involved in the repair of 8-oxoguanine that may result from ROS damage; however no association was found with the risk for malignant mesothelioma [114]. Similarly, no association between this polymorphism and the risk for malignant mesothelioma was observed in a Slovenian study cohort of 150 malignant mesothelioma patients and 122 controls, who were occupationally exposed to asbestos but did not develop any asbestos-related diseases [102].

Recently, a larger number of 273 malignant mesothelioma patients and 193 controls from the same Slovenian cohort were analysed for four SNPs in two DNA repair genes (*ERCC1* rs11615, rs3212986, and *XRCC1* rs1799782, rs25487), but only *ERCC1* rs3212986 was found to be significantly associated with the risk for malignant mesothelioma. However, this polymorphism was found to have a protective effect as carriers of *ERCC1* rs3212986 heterozygous GT or homozygous TT genotypes had a decreased risk of malignant mesothelioma [115].

4. Gene-environment interactions in asbestos-related pleural diseases

It has become increasingly obvious that both environmental and genetic factors may influence the development of many diseases [116–119], including asbestos-related pleural diseases.

Therefore it is important to consider gene-environment interactions when studying diseases related to exposure to different hazards, such as asbestos. Environmental and lifestyle factors have been investigated in many epidemiological studies using self-reported information obtained by questionnaires, interviews, records, or measurements of exposure. However, very few epidemiological studies included the information on genetic risk factors. Similarly, many studies investigating genetic factors obtained little information on environmental factors and lifestyle. Genetic predisposition can be presumed from family history, phenotypic characteristics (e.g., metabolic capacity), or, most importantly, the analysis of DNA sequence. The research into gene-environment interactions requires the information on both environmental and genetic factors [116–118]. Primary candidates for the gene-environment interaction studies have been mostly genes coding for xenobiotic metabolising enzymes. Genetic variability in these genes may lead to interindividual differences in capacity for xenobiotics metabolism, thus modifying an individual's susceptibility to the development of diseases [116]. Furthermore, genetic factors usually do not act independently but may also interact or modify each other. This applies also to asbestos-related pleural diseases [102].

The results of the studies performed so far indicate that in addition to asbestos exposure, the genetic factors, as well as the interactions between genetic factors and asbestos exposure, may have an important impact on the risk of asbestos-related pleural diseases, in particular on malignant mesothelioma [102, 115, 120, 121].

Regarding asbestos-related pleural diseases, the interactions between genetic factors and asbestos exposure have been studied in the case of malignant mesothelioma [102, 115, 120, 121].

The case-control study of Franko et al. investigated the influence of functional polymorphisms of *NQO1*, *CAT*, *SOD2*, and *hOGG1* genes, gene-gene interactions, and gene-environment interactions on malignant mesothelioma risk. The authors reported that although there was no independent association between either *CAT* rs1001179 or *hOGG1* rs1052133 polymorphism and malignant mesothelioma, the interaction between both polymorphisms showed a protective effect. However, no interaction was found between investigated genetic polymorphisms and asbestos exposure [102].

The case-control study of Levpuscek et al. that investigated the influence of functional polymorphisms in *ERCC1* and *XRCC1* genes, the interactions between these polymorphisms, as well as the interactions between these polymorphisms and asbestos exposure on malignant mesothelioma risk found that interaction between *ERCC1* rs11615 polymorphism and asbestos exposure significantly influenced the risk of this cancer. Carriers of polymorphic *ERCC1* rs11615 allele who were exposed to the low level of asbestos had a decreased risk of malignant mesothelioma. Based on these findings, it has been suggested that the genetic variability of DNA repair mechanisms could contribute to the risk of developing of this aggressive cancer [115].

The possible impact of gene-environment interactions on pleural malignant mesothelioma risk was investigated also in the study of Tunesi et al., who conducted a gene-environment interaction analysis including asbestos exposure and 15 single nucleotide polymorphisms (SNPs) previously identified through a genome-wide association study on Italian subjects. Positive deviation from additivity was found for six SNPs (rs1508805, rs2501618, rs4701085, rs4290865, rs10519201, and rs763271), and four of them (rs1508805, rs2501618, rs4701085, and rs10519201) deviated also from multiplicative models. Generalised multifactor dimensionality reduction analysis showed a strong malignant pleural mesothelioma risk due to asbestos exposure and suggested a possible synergistic effect between asbestos exposure and rs1508805, rs2501618, and rs5756444. The results of the presented study also suggested that gene-asbestos interaction may play an additional role in malignant pleural mesothelioma susceptibility [120].

According to our knowledge and the available literature, the influence of gene-environment interactions on the risk of developing other asbestos-related diseases (pleural plaques, diffuse pleural thickening) has not been studied so far.

5. Conclusions

Given that asbestos is still present in the working and living environment all over the world and that pleural asbestos-related diseases, in particular malignant mesothelioma, represent an important health problem worldwide, further research is needed to identify new serum and genetic and epigenetic markers of risk for developing these diseases, for early diagnosis, and for prediction of disease progression and response to treatment. The increasing incidence and poor prognosis of pleural malignant mesothelioma calls for new more effective detection methods, including the identification of novel biomarkers for early and reliable detection of this aggressive cancer, especially in high-risk populations with a known history of asbestos exposure. The influence of gene-environment interactions on the risk of these diseases may be particularly important and should be further investigated. These findings may serve as a basis for the development of new methods for an earlier diagnosis of asbestos-related pleural diseases and may also be used to identify new targets for a more effective treatment, especially of malignant mesothelioma. Furthermore, they could add to our understanding of pathogenesis of asbestos-related pleural diseases and enable their prevention. In this way, they could significantly contribute to the improvement of the quality of life as well as to prolonging lifespan and ageing of subjects exposed to asbestos.

Author details

Vita Dolzan[1]* and Alenka Franko[2]

1 Pharmacogenetics Laboratory, Institute of Biochemistry, Faculty of Medicine, University of Ljubljana, Slovenia

2 Clinical Institute of Occupational Medicine, University Medical Centre, Ljubljana, Slovenia

*Address all correspondence to: vita.dolzan@mf.uni-lj.si

IntechOpen

© 2019 The Author(s). Licensee IntechOpen. This chapter is distributed under the terms of the Creative Commons Attribution License (http://creativecommons.org/licenses/by/3.0), which permits unrestricted use, distribution, and reproduction in any medium, provided the original work is properly cited.

References

[1] Jakobsson K, Stromberg U, Albin M, Welinder H, Hagmar L. Radiological changes in asbestos cement workers. Occupational and Environmental Medicine. 1995;**52**(1):20-27

[2] Hillerdal G, Henderson DW. Asbestos, asbestosis, pleural plaques and lung cancer. Scandinavian Journal of Work, Environment & Health. 1997;**23**(2):93-103

[3] Cugell DW, Kamp DW. Asbestos and the pleura: A review. Chest. 2004;**125**(3):1103-1117

[4] Antao VC, Larson TC, Horton DK. Libby vermiculite exposure and risk of developing asbestos-related lung and pleural diseases. Current Opinion in Pulmonary Medicine. 2012;**18**(2):161-167

[5] Maxim LD, Niebo R, Utell MJ. Are pleural plaques an appropriate endpoint for risk analyses? Inhalation Toxicology. 2015;**27**(7):321-334

[6] Clarke CC, Mowat FS, Kelsh MA, Roberts MA. Pleural plaques: A review of diagnostic issues and possible nonasbestos factors. Archives of Environmental & Occupational Health. 2006;**61**(4):183-192

[7] Solbes E, Harper RW. Biological responses to asbestos inhalation and pathogenesis of asbestos-related benign and malignant disease. Journal of Investigative Medicine. 2018;**66**(4):721-727

[8] Stayner L, Welch LS, Lemen R. The worldwide pandemic of asbestos-related diseases. Annual Review of Public Health. 2013;**34**:205-216

[9] Vainio H. Epidemics of asbestos-related diseases—Something old, something new. Scandinavian Journal of Work, Environment & Health. 2015;**41**(1):1-4. DOI: 10.5271/sjweh.3471. Epub 2014 Dec 4

[10] Marsili D, Terracini B, Santana VS, Ramos-Bonilla JP, Pasetto R, Mazzeo A, et al. Prevention of asbestos-related disease in countries currently using asbestos. International Journal of Environmental Research and Public Health. 2016;**13**(5)

[11] Takahashi K, Landrigan PJ. The global health dimensions of asbestos and asbestos-related diseases. Annals of Global Health. 2016;**82**(1):209-213

[12] Dolzan V, Metoda D-F, Franko A. In: Orhan K, editor. Gene-Environment Interactions: The Case of Asbestosis. Rijeka: InTech; 2017

[13] Visona SD, Villani S, Manzoni F, Chen Y, Ardissino G, Russo F, et al. Impact of asbestos on public health: A retrospective study on a series of subjects with occupational and non-occupational exposure to asbestos during the activity of Fibronit plant (Broni, Italy). Journal of Public Health Research. 2018;**7**(3):20

[14] Diego Roza C, Cruz Carmona MJ, Fernandez Alvarez R, Ferrer Sancho J, Marin Martinez B, Martinez Gonzalez C, et al. Recommendations for the diagnosis and management of asbestos-related pleural and pulmonary disease. Archivos de Bronconeumología. 2017;**53**(8):437-442

[15] Diagnosis and initial management of nonmalignant diseases related to asbestos. American Journal of Respiratory and Critical Care Medicine. 2004;**170**(6):691-715

[16] Clark KA, Flynn JJ 3rd, Karmaus WJJ, Mohr LC. The effects of pleural plaques on longitudinal lung function in vermiculite miners of Libby, Montana. The American Journal of the Medical Sciences. 2017;**353**(6):533-542

[17] Araki T, Yanagawa M, Sun FJ, Dupuis J, Nishino M, Yamada Y, et al. Pleural abnormalities in the Framingham heart study: Prevalence and CT image features. Occupational and Environmental Medicine. 2017;**74**(10):756-761

[18] Larson TC, Lewin M, Gottschall EB, Antao VC, Kapil V, Rose CS. Associations between radiographic findings and spirometry in a community exposed to Libby amphibole. Occupational and Environmental Medicine. 2012;**69**(5):361-366

[19] Kim Y, Myong JP, Lee JK, Kim JS, Kim YK, Jung SH. CT characteristics of pleural plaques related to occupational or environmental asbestos exposure from South Korean asbestos mines. Korean Journal of Radiology. 2015;**16**(5):1142-1152

[20] Mazzei MA, Contorni F, Gentili F, Guerrini S, Mazzei FG, Pinto A, et al. Incidental and underreported pleural plaques at chest CT: Do not miss them-asbestos exposure still exists. BioMed Research International. 2017;**6797826**(10):5

[21] Hansell DM, Bankier AA, MacMahon H, McLoud TC, Muller NL, Remy J. Fleischner Society: Glossary of terms for thoracic imaging. Radiology. 2008;**246**(3):697-722

[22] Dalphin JC. Follow-up of subjects occupationally exposed to asbestos, what are the objectives, the benefits, and the possible risks? Revue des Maladies Respiratoires. 2011;**28**(10):1230-1240

[23] Fishwick D, Barber CM. Non-malignant asbestos-related diseases: A clinical view. Clinical Medicine. 2014;**14**(1):68-71

[24] Ameille J, Brochard P, Letourneux M, Paris C, Pairon JC. Asbestos-related cancer risk in patients with asbestosis or pleural plaques. Revue des Maladies Respiratoires. 2011;**28**(6):008

[25] Hillerdal G. Pleural plaques and risk for bronchial carcinoma and mesothelioma. A prospective study. Chest. 1994;**105**(1):144-150

[26] Karjalainen A, Pukkala E, Kauppinen T, Partanen T. Incidence of cancer among Finnish patients with asbestos-related pulmonary or pleural fibrosis. Cancer Causes & Control. 1999;**10**(1):51-57

[27] Pairon JC, Laurent F, Rinaldo M, Clin B, Andujar P, Ameille J, et al. Pleural plaques and the risk of pleural mesothelioma. Journal of the National Cancer Institute. 2013;**105**(4):293-301

[28] Reid A, de Klerk N, Ambrosini GL, Olsen N, Pang SC, Berry G, et al. The effect of asbestosis on lung cancer risk beyond the dose related effect of asbestos alone. Occupational and Environmental Medicine. 2005;**62**(12):885-889

[29] Fletcher DE. A mortality study of shipyard workers with pleural plaques. British Journal of Industrial Medicine. 1972;**29**(2):142-145

[30] Cullen MR, Barnett MJ, Balmes JR, Cartmel B, Redlich CA, Brodkin CA, et al. Predictors of lung cancer among asbestos-exposed men in the {beta}-carotene and retinol efficacy trial. American Journal of Epidemiology. 2005;**161**(3):260-270

[31] Partanen T, Nurminen M, Zitting A, Koskinen H, Wiikeri M, Ahlman K. Localized pleural plaques and lung cancer. American Journal of Industrial Medicine. 1992;**22**(2):185-192

[32] Ohlson CG, Bodin L, Rydman T, Hogstedt C. Ventilatory decrements in former asbestos cement workers: A four year follow up. British Journal of Industrial Medicine. 1985;**42**(9):612-616

[33] Miller A, Miller JA. Diffuse thickening superimposed on circumscribed pleural thickening related to asbestos exposure. American Journal of Industrial Medicine. 1993;**23**(6):859-871

[34] Rudd RM. New developments in asbestos-related pleural disease. Thorax. 1996;**51**(2):210-216

[35] McLoud TC, Woods BO, Carrington CB, Epler GR, Gaensler EA. Diffuse pleural thickening in an asbestos-exposed population: Prevalence and causes. AJR. American Journal of Roentgenology. 1985;**144**(1):9-18

[36] Copley SJ, Wells AU, Rubens MB, Chabat F, Sheehan RE, Musk AW, et al. Functional consequences of pleural disease evaluated with chest radiography and CT. Radiology. 2001;**220**(1):237-243

[37] de Fonseka D, Edey A, Stadon L, Viner J, Darby M, Maskell NA. The physiological consequences of different distributions of diffuse pleural thickening on CT imaging. The British Journal of Radiology. 2017;**90**(1077):14

[38] Fujimoto N, Kato K, Usami I, Sakai F, Tokuyama T, Hayashi S, et al. Asbestos-related diffuse pleural thickening. Respiration. 2014;**88**(4):277-284

[39] Fujimoto N, Gemba K, Aoe K, Kato K, Yokoyama T, Usami I, et al. Clinical investigation of benign Asbestos pleural effusion. Pulmonary Medicine. 2015;**416179**(10):24

[40] Eisenstadt HB. Asbestos pleurisy. Diseases of the Chest. 1964;**46**:78-81

[41] Arnold DT, De Fonseka D, Perry S, Morley A, Harvey JE, Medford A, et al. Investigating unilateral pleural effusions: The role of cytology. The European Respiratory Journal. 2018;**52**(5):01254-02018

[42] Shehata M, Zaid F, Ottaviano P, Shweihat Y, Munn N. Case report: Steroid responsive mesothelioma-related pleural effusion. Respiratory Medicine Case Reports. 2018 Dec 19;**26**:131-135. DOI: 10.1016/j.rmcr.2018.12.006. eCollection 2019

[43] Sneddon S, Dick I, Lee YCG, Musk AWB, Patch AM, Pearson JV, et al. Malignant cells from pleural fluids in malignant mesothelioma patients reveal novel mutations. Lung Cancer. 2018;**119**:64-70

[44] Robinson BW, Lake RA. Advances in malignant mesothelioma. The New England Journal of Medicine. 2005;**353**(15):1591-1603

[45] King JE, Galateau-Salle F, Hasleton PS. In: O'Byrne K, Rusch V, editors. Malignant Pleural Mesothelioma: Histopathology of Malignant Pleural Mesothelioma. Oxford, New York, Auckland, Cape Town, Hong Kong, Karachi: Oxford University Press; 2006

[46] Rossini M, Rizzo P, Bononi I, Clementz A, Ferrari R, Martini F, et al. New perspectives on diagnosis and therapy of malignant pleural mesothelioma. Frontiers in Oncology. 2018;**8**(91)

[47] McDonald JC, McDonald AD. The epidemiology of mesothelioma in historical context. The European Respiratory Journal. 1996;**9**(9):1932-1942

[48] Franko A, Dolzan V, Kovac V, Arneric N, Dodic-Fikfak M. Soluble mesothelin-related peptides levels in patients with malignant mesothelioma. Disease Markers. 2012;**32**(2):123-131

[49] Bianchi C, Giarelli L, Grandi G, Brollo A, Ramani L, Zuch C. Latency periods in asbestos-related mesothelioma of the pleura. European Journal of Cancer Prevention. 1997;**6**(2):162-166

[50] McElvenny DM, Darnton AJ, Price MJ, Hodgson JT. Mesothelioma mortality in Great Britain from 1968 to 2001. Occupational Medicine. 2005;**55**(2):79-87

[51] Peake MD, Entwisle J, Gray SG. In: O'Byrne K, Rusch V, editors. Malignant Pleural Mesothelioma: Clinical Presentation, Radiological Evaluation and Diagnosis. Oxford, New York, Auckland, Cape Town, Hong Kong, Karachi: Oxford University Press; 2006

[52] Yates DH, Corrin B, Stidolph PN, Browne K. Malignant mesothelioma in south East England: Clinicopathological experience of 272 cases. Thorax. 1997;**52**(6):507-512

[53] Bibby AC, Tsim S, Kanellakis N, Ball H, Talbot DC, Blyth KG, et al. Malignant pleural mesothelioma: An update on investigation, diagnosis and treatment. European Respiratory Review. 2016;**25**(142):472-486

[54] Ribak J, Lilis R, Suzuki Y, Penner L, Selikoff IJ. Malignant mesothelioma in a cohort of asbestos insulation workers: Clinical presentation, diagnosis, and causes of death. British Journal of Industrial Medicine. 1988;**45**(3):182-187

[55] Rusch VW. Diagnosis and treatment of pleural mesothelioma. Seminars in Surgical Oncology. 1990;**6**(5):279-285

[56] Suzuki Y. Pathology of human malignant mesothelioma. Seminars in Oncology. 1981;**8**(3):268-282

[57] Bianco A, Valente T, De Rimini ML, Sica G, Fiorelli A. Clinical diagnosis of malignant pleural mesothelioma. Journal of Thoracic Disease. 2018;**10**(Suppl. 2):S253-SS61

[58] Scherpereel A, Grigoriu B, Conti M, Gey T, Gregoire M, Copin MC, et al. Soluble mesothelin-related peptides in the diagnosis of malignant pleural mesothelioma. American Journal of Respiratory and Critical Care Medicine. 2006;**173**(10):1155-1160

[59] Beyer HL, Geschwindt RD, Glover CL, Tran L, Hellstrom I, Hellstrom KE, et al. MESOMARK: A potential test for malignant pleural mesothelioma. Clinical Chemistry. 2007;**53**(4):666-672

[60] Cristaudo A, Foddis R, Vivaldi A, Guglielmi G, Dipalma N, Filiberti R, et al. Clinical significance of serum mesothelin in patients with mesothelioma and lung cancer. Clinical Cancer Research. 2007;**13**(17):5076-5081

[61] Pass HI, Levin SM, Harbut MR, Melamed J, Chiriboga L, Donington J, et al. Fibulin-3 as a blood and effusion biomarker for pleural mesothelioma. The New England Journal of Medicine. 2012;**367**(15):1417-1427

[62] Kovac V, Dodic-Fikfak M, Arneric N, Dolzan V, Franko A. Fibulin-3 as a biomarker of response to treatment in malignant mesothelioma. Radiology and Oncology. 2015;**49**(3):279-285

[63] Goricar K, Kovac V, Franko A, Dodic-Fikfak M, Dolzan V. Serum survivin levels and outcome of chemotherapy in patients with malignant mesothelioma. Disease Markers. 2015;**316739**(10):16

[64] Rosenzweig KE. Malignant pleural mesothelioma: Adjuvant therapy with radiation therapy. Annals of Translational Medicine. 2017;**5**(11):25

[65] Nowak AK. Chemotherapy for malignant pleural mesothelioma: A review of current management and a look to the future. Annals of Cardiothoracic Surgery. 2012;**1**(4):508-515

[66] Vogelzang NJ, Rusthoven JJ, Symanowski J, Denham C, Kaukel E, Ruffie P, et al. Phase III study of pemetrexed in combination with cisplatin versus cisplatin alone in

patients with malignant pleural mesothelioma. Journal of Clinical Oncology. 2003;**21**(14):2636-2644

[67] Kovac V, Zwitter M, Rajer M, Marin A, Debeljak A, Smrdel U, et al. A phase II trial of low-dose gemcitabine in a prolonged infusion and cisplatin for malignant pleural mesothelioma. Anti-Cancer Drugs. 2012;**23**(2):230-238

[68] Kovac V, Zwitter M, Zagar T. Improved survival after introduction of chemotherapy for malignant pleural mesothelioma in Slovenia: Population-based survey of 444 patients. Radiology and Oncology. 2012;**46**(2):136-144

[69] Lee CW, Murray N, Anderson H, Rao SC, Bishop W. Outcomes with first-line platinum-based combination chemotherapy for malignant pleural mesothelioma: A review of practice in British Columbia. Lung Cancer. 2009;**64**(3):308-313

[70] Ak G, Metintas S, Akarsu M, Metintas M. The effectiveness and safety of platinum-based pemetrexed and platinum-based gemcitabine treatment in patients with malignant pleural mesothelioma. BMC Cancer. 2015;**15**(510):015-1519

[71] Becklake MR. Exposure to asbestos and human disease. The New England Journal of Medicine. 1982;**306**(24):1480-1482. DOI: 10.1056/NEJM198206173062409

[72] Craighead JE, Mossman BT. The pathogenesis of asbestos-associated diseases. The New England Journal of Medicine. 1982;**306**(24):1446-1455

[73] Nishimura SL, Broaddus VC. Asbestos-induced pleural disease. Clinics in Chest Medicine. 1998;**19**(2):311-329

[74] Abratt RP, Vorobiof DA, White N. Asbestos and mesothelioma in South Africa. Lung Cancer. 2004;**45**(1):007

[75] Wagner GR et al. . In: Rosenstock L, Mark C, Brodkin CA, Redlich CA, editors. Mineral Dust: Asbestos, Silica, Coal, Manufactured Fibers. 2nd ed. Elsevier Saunders: Philadelphia, Edinburgh, New York, St Louis, Sydney, Toronto; 2005

[76] IARC. Asbestos. IARC Working Group: Lyon; 1972

[77] IARC. IARC Monographs on the Evaluation of Carcinogenic Risk of Chemicals to Man. Some Inorganic and Organometalic Compounds. Lyon: International Agency for Research on Cancer; 1973

[78] Mossman BT. Mechanisms of asbestos carcinogenesis and toxicity: The amphibole hypothesis revisited. British Journal of Industrial Medicine. 1993;**50**(8):673-676. DOI: 10.1136/oem.50.8.673

[79] Piolatto G, Negri E, La Vecchia C, Pira E, Decarli A, Peto J. An update of cancer mortality among chrysotile asbestos miners in Balangero, northern Italy. British Journal of Industrial Medicine. 1990;**47**(12):810-814

[80] Guthrie GD Jr. Mineral properties and their contributions to particle toxicity. Environmental Health Perspectives. 1997;**5**:1003-1011

[81] Dodic Fikfak M, Kriebel D, Quinn MM, Eisen EA, Wegman DH. A case control study of lung cancer and exposure to chrysotile and amphibole at a Slovenian asbestos-cement plant. The Annals of Occupational Hygiene. 2007;**51**(3):261-268

[82] Brodkin CA, Rosenstock L. Asbestos and Asbestos-Related Pleural Disease. In: Rosenstock L, Cullen M, Brodkin CA, Redlich CA, editors. 2nd ed. Elsevier Saunders: Philadelphia, Edinburgh, New York, St Louis, Sydney, Toronto; 2005

[83] Rom W. In: Rom WN, editor. Asbestosis, Pleural Fibrosis, and Lung Cancer. 4th ed. Wolters Kluwer, Lippincott Williams & Wilkins: Philadelphia, Baltimore, New York, London, Buenos Aires, Hong Kong, Sydney, Tokyo; 2007

[84] Liu G, Cheresh P, Kamp DW. Molecular basis of asbestos-induced lung disease. Annual Review of Pathology. 2013;**8**:161-187

[85] Gilmour PS, Brown DM, Beswick PH, MacNee W, Rahman I, Donaldson K. Free radical activity of industrial fibers: Role of iron in oxidative stress and activation of transcription factors. Environmental Health Perspectives. 1997;**5**:1313-1317

[86] Chew SH, Toyokuni S. Malignant mesothelioma as an oxidative stress-induced cancer: An update. Free Radical Biology & Medicine. 2015;**86**:166-178

[87] Sayan M, Mossman BT. The NLRP3 inflammasome in pathogenic particle and fibre-associated lung inflammation and diseases. Particle and Fibre Toxicology. 2016;**13**(1):016-0162

[88] Yang H, Rivera Z, Jube S, Nasu M, Bertino P, Goparaju C, et al. Programmed necrosis induced by asbestos in human mesothelial cells causes high-mobility group box 1 protein release and resultant inflammation. Proceedings of the National Academy of Sciences of the United States of America. 2010;**107**(28):12611-12616

[89] Kadariya Y, Menges CW, Talarchek J, Cai KQ, Klein-Szanto AJ, Pietrofesa RA, et al. Inflammation-related IL1beta/IL1R signaling promotes the development of asbestos-induced malignant mesothelioma. Cancer Prevention Research. 2016;**9**(5):406-414

[90] Helmig S, Belwe A, Schneider J. Association of transforming growth factor beta1 gene polymorphisms and asbestos-induced fibrosis and tumors. Journal of Investigative Medicine. 2009;**57**(5):655-661

[91] Helmig S, Aliahmadi N, Schneider J. Tumour necrosis factor-alpha gene polymorphisms in asbestos-induced diseases. Biomarkers. 2010;**15**(5):400-409

[92] Lagente V, Manoury B, Nenan S, Le Quement C, Martin-Chouly C, Boichot E. Role of matrix metalloproteinases in the development of airway inflammation and remodeling. Brazilian Journal of Medical and Biological Research. 2005;**38**(10):1521-1530

[93] Mossman BT, Shukla A, Heintz NH, Verschraegen CF, Thomas A, Hassan R. New insights into understanding the mechanisms, pathogenesis, and management of malignant mesotheliomas. The American Journal of Pathology. 2013;**182**(4):1065-1077

[94] Huang SX, Jaurand MC, Kamp DW, Whysner J, Hei TK. Role of mutagenicity in asbestos fiber-induced carcinogenicity and other diseases. Journal of Toxicology and Environmental Health. Part B, Critical Reviews. 2011;**14**(1-4):179-245

[95] Bononi A, Napolitano A, Pass HI, Yang H, Carbone M. Latest developments in our understanding of the pathogenesis of mesothelioma and the design of targeted therapies. Expert Review of Respiratory Medicine. 2015;**9**(5):633-654

[96] Hayes JD, Flanagan JU, Jowsey IR. Glutathione transferases. Annual Review of Pharmacology and Toxicology. 2005;**45**:51-88

[97] Hein DW. Molecular genetics and function of NAT1 and NAT2: Role in aromatic amine metabolism and carcinogenesis. Mutation Research. 2002;**507**:65-77

[98] Hirvonen A, Tuimala J, Ollikainen T, Linnainmaa K, Kinnula V. Manganese superoxide dismutase genotypes and asbestos-associated pulmonary disorders. Cancer Letters. 2002;**178**(1):71-74

[99] Kinnula VL, Torkkeli T, Kristo P, Sormunen R, Soini Y, Paakko P, et al. Ultrastructural and chromosomal studies on manganese superoxide dismutase in malignant mesothelioma. American Journal of Respiratory Cell and Molecular Biology. 2004;**31**(2):147-153

[100] Landi S, Gemignani F, Neri M, Barale R, Bonassi S, Bottari F, et al. Polymorphisms of glutathione-S-transferase M1 and manganese superoxide dismutase are associated with the risk of malignant pleural mesothelioma. International Journal of Cancer. 2007;**120**(12):2739-2743

[101] Kukkonen MK, Hamalainen S, Kaleva S, Vehmas T, Huuskonen MS, Oksa P, et al. Genetic susceptibility to asbestos-related fibrotic pleuropulmonary changes. The European Respiratory Journal. 2011;**38**(3):672-678

[102] Franko A, Kotnik N, Goricar K, Kovac V, Dodic-Fikfak M, Dolzan V. The influence of genetic variability on the risk of developing malignant mesothelioma. Radiology and Oncology. 2018;**52**(1):105-111

[103] Hirvonen A, Pelin K, Tammilehto L, Karjalainen A, Mattson K, Linnainmaa K. Inherited GSTM1 and NAT2 defects as concurrent risk modifiers in asbestos-related human malignant mesothelioma. Cancer Research. 1995;**55**(14):2981-2983

[104] Hirvonen A, Saarikoski ST, Linnainmaa K, Koskinen K, Husgafvel-Pursiainen K, Mattson K, et al. Glutathione S-transferase and N-acetyltransferase genotypes and asbestos-associated pulmonary disorders. Journal of the National Cancer Institute. 1996;**88**(24):1853-1856

[105] Neri M, Taioli E, Filiberti R, Paolo Ivaldi G, Aldo Canessa P, Verna A, et al. Metabolic genotypes as modulators of asbestos-related pleural malignant mesothelioma risk: A comparison of Finnish and Italian populations. International Journal of Hygiene and Environmental Health. 2006;**209**(4):393-398

[106] Fretland AJ, Omiecinski CJ. Epoxide hydrolases: Biochemistry and molecular biology. Chemico-Biological Interactions. 2000;**129**(1-2):41-59

[107] Kukkonen MK, Vehmas T, Piirila P, Hirvonen A. Genes involved in innate immunity associated with asbestos-related fibrotic changes. Occupational and Environmental Medicine. 2014;**71**(1):48-54

[108] Verma D, Lerm M, Blomgran Julinder R, Eriksson P, Soderkvist P, Sarndahl E. Gene polymorphisms in the NALP3 inflammasome are associated with interleukin-1 production and severe inflammation: Relation to common inflammatory diseases? Arthritis and Rheumatism. 2008;**58**(3):888-894

[109] Wilson AG, Symons JA, McDowell TL, McDevitt HO, Duff GW. Effects of a polymorphism in the human tumor necrosis factor alpha promoter on transcriptional activation. Proceedings of the National Academy of Sciences of the United States of America. 1997;**94**(7):3195-3199

[110] Grainger DJ, Heathcote K, Chiano M, Snieder H, Kemp PR, Metcalfe JC, et al. Genetic control of the circulating concentration of transforming growth factor type beta1. Human Molecular Genetics. 1999;**8**(1):93-97

[111] Strbac D, Goricar K, Dolzan V, Kovac V. Matrix metalloproteinases

polymorphisms as baseline risk predictors in malignant pleural mesothelioma. Radiology and Oncology. 2018;**52**(2):160-166

[112] Strbac D, Goricar K, Dolzan V, Kovac V. Matrix metalloproteinases polymorphisms as prognostic biomarkers in malignant pleural mesothelioma. Disease Markers. 2017;**8069529**(10):12

[113] Dianzani I, Gibello L, Biava A, Giordano M, Bertolotti M, Betti M, et al. Polymorphisms in DNA repair genes as risk factors for asbestos-related malignant mesothelioma in a general population study. Mutation Research. 2006;**599**(1-2):124-134

[114] Betti M, Ferrante D, Padoan M, Guarrera S, Giordano M, Aspesi A, et al. XRCC1 and ERCC1 variants modify malignant mesothelioma risk: A case-control study. Mutation Research. 2011;**708**(1-2):11-20

[115] Levpuscek K, Goricar K, Kovac V, Dolzan V, Franko A. The influence of genetic variability of DNA repair mechanisms on the risk of malignant mesothelioma. Radiology and Oncology. 2019;**53**(5):206-212

[116] Mucci LA, Wedren S, Tamimi RM, Trichopoulos D, Adami HO. The role of gene-environment interaction in the aetiology of human cancer: Examples from cancers of the large bowel, lung and breast. Journal of Internal Medicine. 2001;**249**(6):477-493

[117] Boks MP, Schipper M, Schubart CD, Sommer IE, Kahn RS, Ophoff RA. Investigating gene environment interaction in complex diseases: Increasing power by selective sampling for environmental exposure. International Journal of Epidemiology. 2007;**36**(6):1363-1369

[118] Hunter DJ. Gene-environment interactions in human diseases. Nature Reviews. Genetics. 2005;**6**(4):287-298

[119] Rothman KJ, Greenland S, Poole C, Lash TL. In: Rothman KJ, Greenland S, Lash TL, editors. Causation and Cause Inference. Philadelphia, Baltimore, New York, London, Buenos Aires, Hong Kong, Sydney, Tokyo: Lippincott-Raven; 2008

[120] Tunesi S, Ferrante D, Mirabelli D, Andorno S, Betti M, Fiorito G, et al. Gene-asbestos interaction in malignant pleural mesothelioma susceptibility. Carcinogenesis. 2015;**36**(10):1129-1135

[121] Senk B, Goricar K, Kovac V, Dolzan V, Franko A. Genetic polymorphisms in aquaporin 1 as risk factors for malignant mesothelioma and biomarkers of response to cisplatin treatment. Radiology and Oncology. 2019;**53**(1):96-104

Chapter 3

Cosmetic Talcum Powder as a Causative Factor in the Development of Diseases of the Pleura

Ronald E. Gordon

Abstract

This chapter describes some of what is known about the effects of talc as cosmetic or pharmaceutical talcum powder on the pleura and other organs of the human body. It further describes some of the already known mechanisms of how it interacts with human cells and tissue to cause diseases, specifically in the pleura. The effects of talcum powder are well established that the range of diseases include clinical or subclinical inflammation, granulomatous disease and tumors, in the pleura mainly mesotheliomas. Also included are some preliminary evidence indicating what happens in vitro with macrophages in response to talc morphologically and the consequences following the treatment with the release of factors such as chemokines, cytokines and oxidants.

Keywords: cosmetic talcum powder, pleura, granulomas, mesothelioma, lung cancer, asbestos

1. Introduction

It has been demonstrated that both asbestos and talc can and does cause diseases of the pleura [1–9]. Asbestos has been shown to cause the development of benign lesions in pleura termed pleura plaques [10]. These plaques have become a hallmark for asbestos exposure [10–12]. These lesions correlated with interstitial fibrosis of the lung parenchyma [2] and the development of lung tumors [13]. These lesions allow for attribution of asbestos as a causative factor in the development of lung tumors in the absence of interstitial fibrosis [12]. Pleural plaques is also a lesion that indicates asbestos exposure in the absence of interstitial fibrosis and/or lung tumors [12]. Asbestos has been shown to be the cause of tumors of the pleural lining, mesotheliomas [2]. It has been shown that mesotheliomas in men were mostly seen in those men with occupational histories of exposure to asbestos [14]. Similarly, it was demonstrated that the wives of these men that were exposed and women that worked with asbestos also developed the pleural plaques, interstitial fibrosis and mesotheliomas [4, 8, 15, 16]. It was understandable how the asbestos caused the lesions in the pleura of women working with the asbestos, however, it was not initially understood how the wives or children of workers developed these lesions until investigators looked at the clothing of the husbands and determined that they were bringing the asbestos home and the wives or children were exposed cleaning their clothes [15, 16]. However, only about 30% of all the mesotheliomas found in women could be attributed to exposure to asbestos [17]. The remainder of women with mesotheliomas were considered idiopathic because they could not be attributed to a specific asbestos exposure.

With that in mind, I will turn to talc as a cause of pleural diseases. It has been shown that talc causes pneumoconiosis [1]. In some people exposed to talc via inhalation, they have been shown to develop granulomatous lesions in the lung [1]. It was determined that these lesions were developed from a macrophage response directly due to the talc by finding the talc with the macrophages and giant cells in the lesions [18]. Based on the knowledge that the talc will cause a granulomatous reaction with fibrosis, pharmaceutical talc was being used in patients with pleural mesotheliomas who developed pleural effusions. The patients almost always developed pleural effusions with pleural mesotheliomas which had to be drained frequently. It was then determined and that by injecting the pharmaceutical talc into the pleural space, it would insight a granulomatous response which would fill the space between the visceral and parietal pleura with a granulomatous response followed by fibrosis alleviating the need to drain this fluid [19]. This occurred in 100% of the individuals that the talc was injected, as compared with a very low percentage of people getting talc granulomas from breathing talc [19].

It is the purpose of this chapter to further describe the effects of talc, particularly cosmetic talcum powders in the causation of diseases of the pleura. This includes the development of pleura plaques, granulomas and mesotheliomas.

2. Background

It is important to understand how foreign materials such as cosmetic talcum powder can get to the pleura to cause diseases. For the particles contained in the cosmetic talcum powder to get to the pleura under normal circumstances after inhalation would be that these particles are phagocytized by macrophages of the lung and these macrophages enter the lymphatic system and are carried in two directions based on the drainage of the lymphatic system of the lung [20]. The macrophages are carried to the regional lymph nodes along the respiratory bronchial tree and up along the trachea. Alternatively, the lymph drains to the pleura. Another route, although not as good in distributing to the pleura is if the macrophages should enter the blood stream, mainly into the capillaries of the alveolar septa, at the peripheral gas exchange surfaces of the lung [20]. Under those situations, the talc can be taken anywhere in the body. The last way is that it is injected directly into the pleura, termed pleurodesis [21].

Once in the lung, lymph nodes or pleura, the particles induce reactions within cells which result in the production of cytokines, chemokines and oxidants, all of which are responsible for the inducing an inflammatory response and the mechanistic steps in the process of compensated healing or fibrosis [21]. The size of the talc particles appear to be critical to the type of response the cells and the tissue mount [22]. The particle size of cosmetic talc is significantly smaller than that used for talc pleurodesis and therefore the response is very different [22]. The inhalation or injection of this smaller cosmetic talc has a much greater detrimental effect by the inflammatory response it elicits [22].

Similarly, these same cells produce oxidants following activation by the presence of the components of the cosmetic talc powder in addition to producing cytokines, chemokines, IL-6 & 8; TGF-beta, which attract inflammatory cells as well as cells that produce fibrosis [23]. Oxidants are extremely reactive and have the ability to do significant damage to resident cells to cause injury to cells, stress the cells, and cause DNA damage [24]. Such DNA damage can and will cause mutations which can result in cancer development [24]. However, the release of chemokines which stimulate and attract other inflammatory cells, neutrophils, which further release similar factors as the macrophages and but most importantly, additional oxidants. Such mechanisms of injury has been shown over and over again to correlate with the development of cancer, specifically, the resident cells and therefore mesotheliomas [25]. These mesotheliomas in response to the talc has been attributed to contaminating asbestos [25–27]. However, in all the studies, whether looking at mortalities and percentage of mesotheliomas based on exposure to talc or epidemiological studies, there have been none in the past that actually put together all the components of age, sex, amount of exposure and documentation of tissue digestions of lungs, respiratory lymph nodes or abdominal organs, including ovaries to attribute the finding of talc and/or asbestos together. Therefore, it is difficult to conclude that asbestos was the only contributing factor. The talc may well be a contributing factor in both the development of the pleural plaques, mesotheliomas and abdominal mesotheliomas and ovarian cancers.

3. Common cases

The author has now had the opportunity to evaluate approximately 100 plus cases of mesothelioma, pleural and abdominal, of both men and women with only a history of exposure to cosmetic talcum powder, some with exposure to a single cosmetic powder and others to multiple types. However, none of these patients have indicated, based on extensive histories, that there was exposure to occupational or para-occupational to a commercial asbestos or products containing added asbestos. There are a few cases where there may have been brief, single exposures to possible sources of products that may have contained asbestos. It is important to emphasize “brief” as compared to everyday if not multiple times per day exposure to cosmetic talcum powder. The logic only reflects that the cosmetic talcum powder would represent the overall, great majority of particles and fibers found in the lungs and lymph nodes in these patients and would dictate the source of these structures would be from the cosmetic talc rather than the brief potential exposure to another questionable unproven source. The findings of digestions of the lungs and the lymph nodes of the patients show basically all the same structures. Some of the cases are reported as a case study, which is currently under review. One study where that has been published describes the case and what was found in the digested tissue as well as the testing of the cosmetic talc and to correlate it with the potential to breathe both the asbestos fibers and the talc [28]. All of the patients have talc particles, aluminum silicates, some with magnesium, some with iron and some with both. There can also be silica crystals and fibers, silica, talc and aluminum silicates. Further, most of the patients also have asbestos fibers, primarily anthophyllite and tremolite. Even though it has been shown that many of the cosmetic talcum powder containers sold by at least one company also contained chrysotile type asbestos the chrysotile was never found. Based on the ability of the human cells to break the chrysotile down and dissolve it and or move it out of the initial sites, it would not be found in digestions done many years after exposure. The presence of either type of asbestos or both are reflective of the types and time frame of the cosmetic talcum powder used. The source of the talcum powder, meaning the mine source and location of the talc may result in the presence of the particles and fibers that contaminate the cosmetic talcum powders as it solidified millions of years before. It is not uncommon that over many years of use and exposure that it is possible for such exposures to be from multiple sources, mines. Therefore, it is not uncommon to find all of the particles and fibers present in most of these patients.

It is important to address the issue of what has been termed intergrowths. Some asbestos analysis laboratories do not confirm or report fibers that can be termed intergrowths. These intergrowths are attributed mostly to anthophyllite fibers. The most common source of such intergrowths has frequently been stated in courts across our country by lawyers and their expert witnesses that suggest the only source of these intergrowths occur where anthophyllite veins meet with talc deposits. This can be true, but more commonly talc is an integral component of anthophyllite all the time [29]. If a mineralogist looks at anthophyllite fibers by what has been termed zone-axis analyses where the anthophyllite is analyzed by tilting and rotating to find possible co-mingling of some talc with the anthophyllite and therefore making the false claim that it is an intergrowth making the fiber non-asbestos. This is also true for transitional fibers because portions of the fibers are anthophyllite. If that portion of the fiber is broken off there would be no way to distinguish it from any other frank anthophyllite fiber. However, it could be interpreted that the combination of primarily an anthophyllite fiber with the talc between the fibrils may be the perfect carcinogen based on action of both types of crystalline structures being present. It is also based on their abilities to cause inflammation by release of chemokines, the development of fibrosis by the release of cytokines and the development of cancer by direct mutation or the production of oxidants which can cause injury or mutation. Therefore, in spite of the fact that most every asbestos analysis laboratory uses selected area electron diffraction (SAED) as the gold standard for defining asbestos type and distinguishing it from a nonasbestos fibers, in this particular case, spending hours manipulating a fiber to show it may have a talc component is a ridiculous exercise knowing that the primary features of this structure represent an anthophyllite fiber and even if it has a small talc component, from a biologic standpoint the cell will see it as an anthophyllite asbestos fiber. This entire concept of an intergrowth is just detraction of reality by a laboratory trying to, in most cases, satisfy a defendant company trying to misrepresent other laboratory findings. However, from a mineralogic standpoint they are fine attributing such a fiber to that of an intergrowth, but it should never be excluded from being called an anthophyllite asbestos fiber. Therefore, the combination of morphology, EDS and flat plane SAED is sufficient to identify an anthophyllite fiber for the purposes of asbestos analysis in human tissues.

There have been many studies linking the use of cosmetic talc and the development of both mesotheliomas, plural and abdominal and ovarian cancer [10, 13, 30, 31]. Most of these studies are based on the patients' reporting significant exposure to cosmetic talcum powder and no exposure to any other asbestos containing product. This leads us to two additional issues that have yet to be resolved: (1) Was the cosmetic talcum powder adequately contaminated with asbestos for the asbestos to be the causative factor all on its own or does the talc itself contribute to the process of tumor development? (2) In the past, there has been an extremely high rate of mesotheliomas in women, as much as 70%, that have been termed idiopathic. Clearly these women when questioned about their medical histories have indicated no evidence or history of asbestos exposure. However, it has become clear that in the past most physicians were not considering cosmetic talcum powder an asbestos product nor were they considering it a source of asbestos that would account for the development of a mesothelioma. Yet again, that appears to exclude the talc itself or its other contaminating components such as fibrous and platy aluminum silicates and fibrous and crystalline silica particles.

To support this concept that other components in the talcum powder may be carcinogenic, are reports attributing fibrous aluminum silicates to the development of mesotheliomas in the form of algorskite (palygorskite) [32]. We already know and understand how talc, silica and aluminum silicates can cause the development of granulomas in the lungs and GI tracts of humans. This again is an inflammatory/immunologic mechanism predominantly in patients that are genetically predisposed. However, predisposed or not if these particles are in a large enough concentration it will produce these inflammatory responses in 100% of the patients. This type of reaction is now well documented as a contributing factor to the development of cancer as a promoter, but possibly as a carcinogen or co-carcinogen as well.

4. Preliminary evidence

With the above in mind, this author has looked directly at the interaction of the particles present in cosmetic talcum powder taken from a container previous extensively tested for the presence of asbestos, tremolite; anthophyllite; and chrysotile, and which no asbestos was found. The experiment was designed to put the cosmetic talc at a very low concentration 0.001 grams per ml distilled water into primary macrophage control cultures differentiated from human blood monocytes. The macrophages were cultured with the cosmetic talcum powder for 12, 24 hours and 3 days. At that point the cultures were fixed with glutaraldehyde and duplicate dishes were processed for observation by scanning electron microscopy (SEM) on the cover slips and the other dish was rubber policed to yield a cell pellet so it could be routinely processed for embedding in epon, ultrathin sectioned double stained and observed by transmission electron microscopy (TEM). The SEM allowed me to determine how the macrophages were collecting and engulfing the particles. The TEM made it possible to see in what structures the particles were contained and how the particles were interacting with the macrophage organelles and how they differ from normal differentiated macrophages.

The results of this preliminary study show that the macrophages engulf/phagocytize the particles (**Figure 1**). In many instances, the particles are just too large for the cells to completely engulf and they extend out of the cell (**Figure 2**). If these

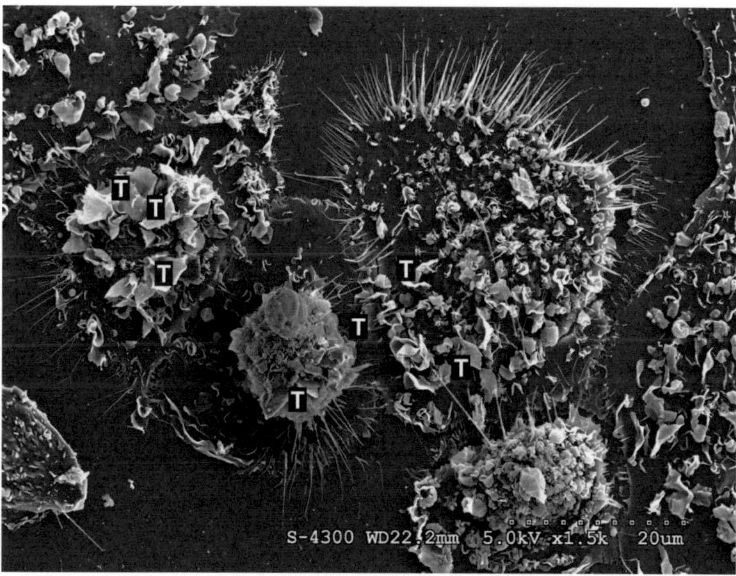

Figure 1.
Scanning electron micrograph (SEM) of a cultured human monocytes differentiated in macrophages collecting and engulfing the talc particles (T).

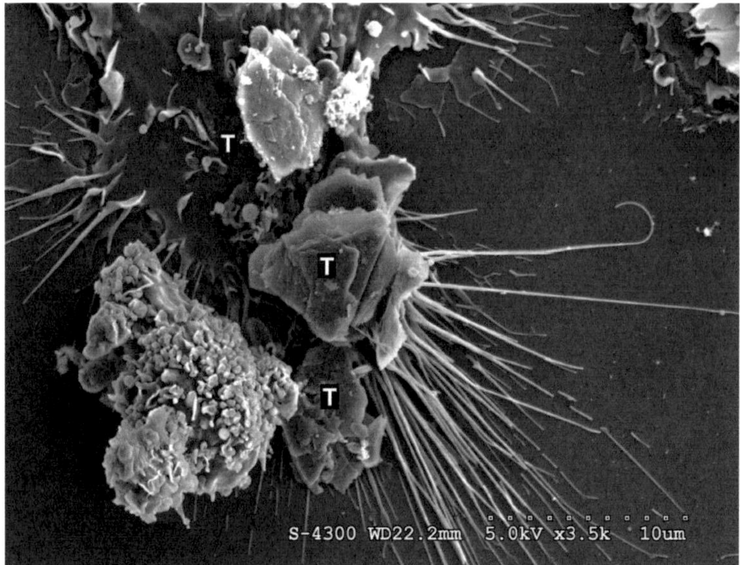

Figure 2.
This SEM shows a cell after 3 days with talc (T) and the particle cannot be completely engulfed in the cell. During this process it is possible to see how intracellular molecules such as the chemokines, cytokines and oxidants can easily leak around the particles outside the cell.

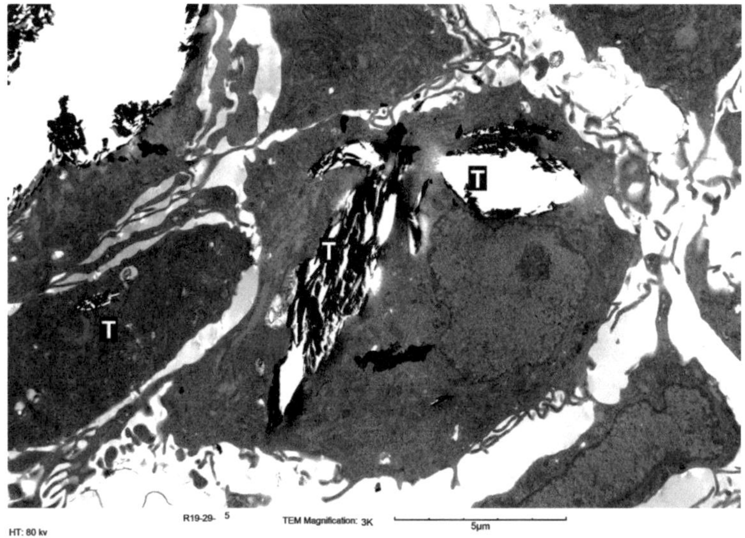

Figure 3.
In this transmission electron micrograph (TEM), it is possible to see the talc particle within the cell. However, because the section of the cell is so thin, it is not possible to determine if the particle has been completely engulfed or not. However, based on what was visualized by SEM, it is likely that the larger talc (T) particles are not completely engulfed.

cells are observed in thin sections by transmission electron microscopy (TEM) it is difficult to determine if the particles are completely within the cells or partially in and partially outside (**Figure 3**). This is similar to what is seen with asbestos fibers that are longer than 10 micrometers. This is very much like inflammatory cell attempting to phagocytize deposits in the kidney glomeruli and just cannot because the deposits are in the basement membrane. This is termed frustrated phagacytosis and results in the leakage of lysosomal enzymes and many other chemokines,

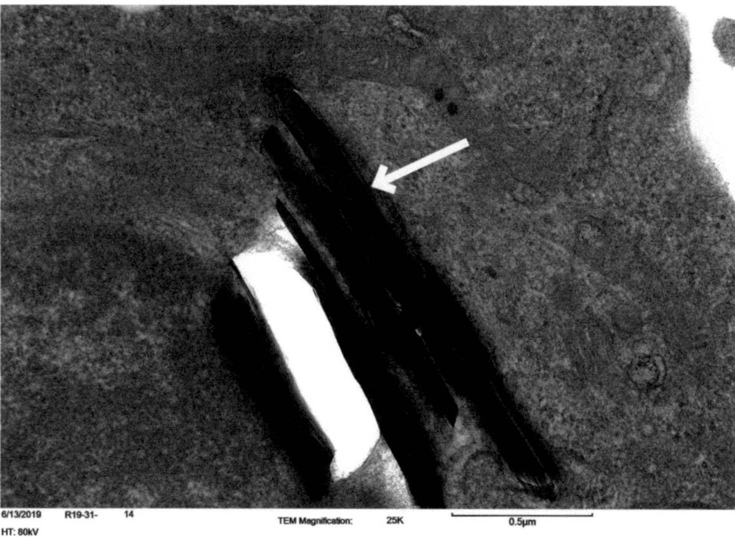

Figure 4.
Normally anything that is endocytosed by macrophages or phagocytic cells are surrounded by the plasma membrane as it endocytoses something. What is very interesting with the talc is that there is no complete membrane surrounding the particle. The membrane is discontinuous within the cell (arrow).

cytokines and oxidants from the macrophages. TEM analysis of the cells exhibited particles in the cytoplasm of the cells and they were not completely enclosed by a single membrane in the 12, 24 or 72 hours specimen (**Figure 4**). The most interesting finding is that these particles as they break down within the cell cytoplasms due to enzyme activity or not do not exhibit being membrane bound (**Figures 5A**, **B**). Remnants of membrane, presumably plasma membranes, can be seen but the talc particles are found mostly free in the cytoplasm of these cells (**Figures 5A**, **B**). It was possible to see smaller particles completely engulfed into the cell that were free, not membrane bound (**Figure 6**). These particles can be seen very close to the nucleus of the cell making direct mechanical interaction with or without cell division possible (**Figure 7**). The significance of this has very detrimental implications for alterations of cellular function. If and when these particles enter mesothelial cells or even lung cells and are free to interact with surrounding organelles and other cellular components, the cells may be stimulated to divide and in doing so during division the chromosomes and DNA are exposed to these particles which can alter the DNA and chromosomes mechanically by charge distribution or any other mechanism including direct oxidant injury to the DNA. This can lead to mutations that will lead or result in the development of tumors.

Support for the morphologic criteria is the biochemical and immunologic criteria showing that cytokines, chemokines and oxidants are released in response to the frustrated phagocytosis. **Figures 8** and **9** support the cytokine up regulation. These are similar, if not exactly the same criteria that had been reported for the interaction of asbestos fibers and macrophages over the years. Based on these preliminary in vitro results, it is not a far reach to implicate talc and its contaminating silica and aluminum silicates as a causative agent in the development of mesotheliomas, lung tumors, gastrointestinal tumors, and ovarian tumors.

Further, the proof of these basic facts and the epidemiologic study of cases that this author has done of asbestos fiber and particle analyses on over 200 cases of men and women who have only exposure to talcum powder with no exposure to any other source of asbestos, and have developed mesotheliomas, pleural and abdominal, and ovarian cancer of epithelial origin. It should be noted here that the

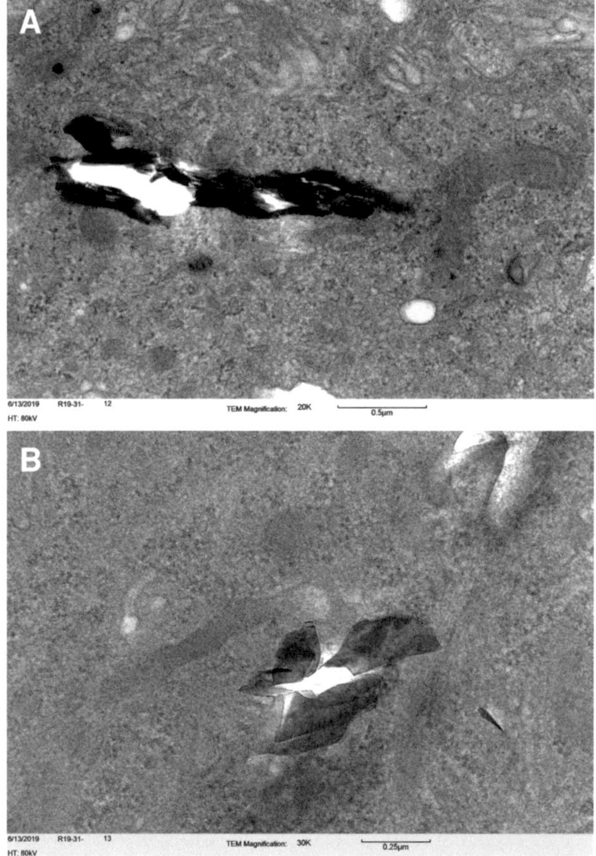

Figure 5.
(A and B) When one observes even the smaller particles that are presumed to be completely within the cell, it is not possible to identify a complete membrane surrounding the particles. It appears that the particles unlike other components taken up by cells, these apparently can be found naked in the cytoplasm.

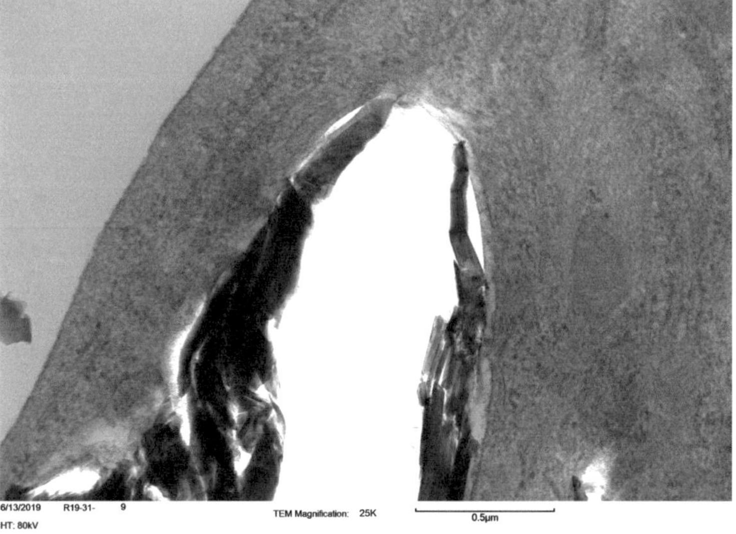

Figure 6.
The larger particles clearly exhibit an absence of membrane and it presence in the cytoplasm where lysosomes and other molecules within the cell can directly interact with the talc particles causing injury to the and leaking components into the media in this case or in tissue to adjacent cells.

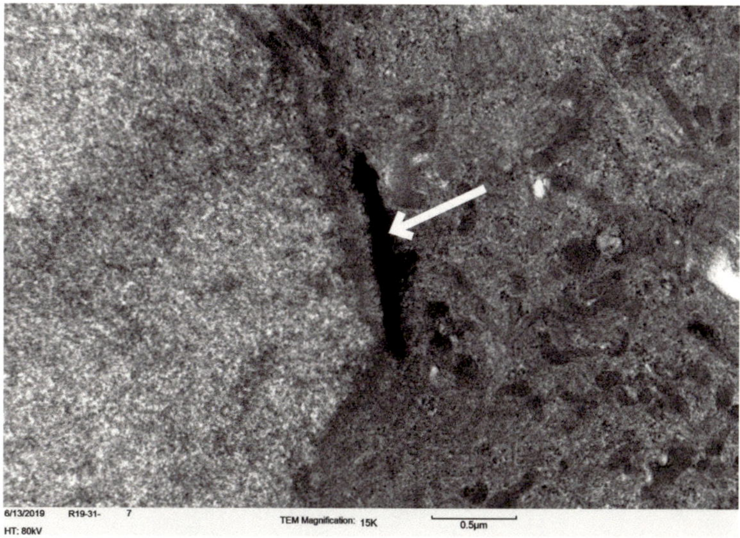

Figure 7.
These small particles and possibly even the larger particles make their way right to the nucleus (arrow).

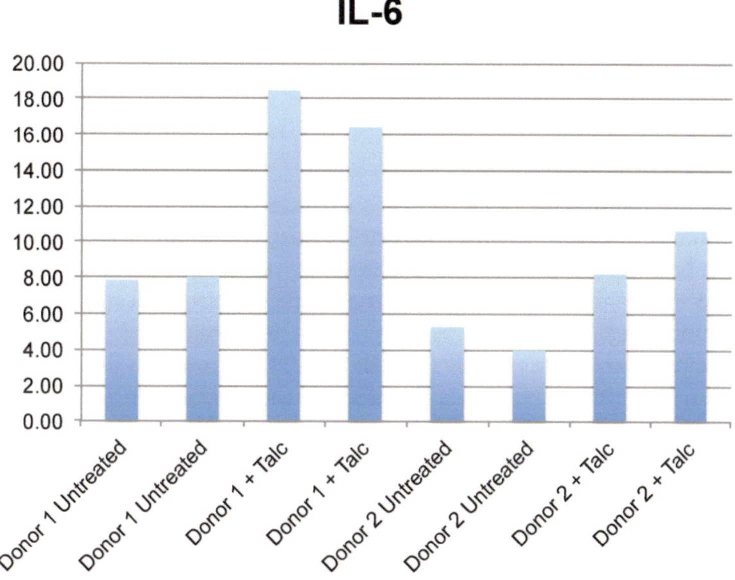

Figure 8.
This is a bar graph exhibiting the results of the IL-6 measurements from the 2 patients under the 3 conditions of control, cultures without talc and with talc added.

outer lining of the ovaries that give rise to the tumors are basically mesothelial cells, just on the surface of ovaries. The correlation of finding significant amounts of talc, aluminum silicates, crystalline silica and in more than half the cases asbestos fibers as compared to background controls with none of the fibers and particles discussed above, supports the concept that cosmetic talcum powder is the causative factor in the development of the mesotheliomas and ovarian cancer. This applies to both abdominal, pleural and ovarian cancer, however, the abdominal mesotheliomas and ovarian cancer represent a cleaner model since analyses of lung and pulmonary lymph nodes frequently contain some talc, aluminum silicates and crystalline silica from the environment and nonasbestos containing materials. However, these

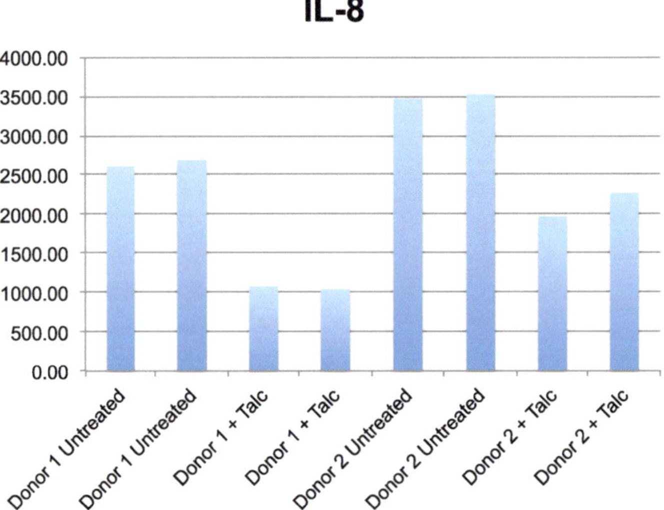

Figure 9.
This is a bar graph exhibiting the results of the IL-8 measurements from the 2 patients under the 3 conditions of control, cultures without talc and with talc added.

components are in relatively small quantities as compared to those individuals that have used cosmetic talcum powder on a regular basis.

5. Summary

There is now significant growing evidence based on basic scientific studies and epidemiologic studies of those patients exposed to cosmetic talcum powders on a regular basis with correlation of isolation of talcum powder components in significantly greater concentration than the contaminating asbestos, that the talc or other aluminum silicate components found in high concentration in the talcum powders strongly implicate the talc itself as a causative factor in the development of all the same lesions: granulomas, fibrosis and tumors, as seen with asbestos. Due to the relatively small amount or absence of an iron oxidant component in the talc and aluminum silicates, it is likely that without a tremendous load the detrimental effects may take years to develop in patients that are predisposed genetically to the actions of these talc particles. This phenomenon may be very much correlated to the development of similar lesions by chrysotile asbestos, having a longer latency from that of commercial amphiboles amosite and crocidolite.

Author details

Ronald E. Gordon
Department of Pathology, Icahn School of Medicine at Mt. Sinai, New York, United States

*Address all correspondence to: ronald.gordon@mountsinai.org

IntechOpen

© 2019 The Author(s). Licensee IntechOpen. This chapter is distributed under the terms of the Creative Commons Attribution License (http://creativecommons.org/licenses/by/3.0), which permits unrestricted use, distribution, and reproduction in any medium, provided the original work is properly cited. CC BY

References

[1] Gibb AE, Pooley FD, Griffiths DM, Mitha R, Craighead JE, Ruttner JR. Talc pneumoconiosis: Apathologic and mineralogic study. Human Pathology. 1991;**23**:1344-1354

[2] Straif K, Benbrahim-Tallaa L, Baan R, et al. A review of human carcinogens--Part C: Metals, arsenic, dusts, and fibres. The Lancet Oncology. 2009;**10**(5):453-454

[3] Wagner JC, Sleggs CA, Marchand P. Diffuse pleural mesothelioma and asbestos exposure in the North Western Cape Province. Occupational and Environmental Medicine. 1960;**17**(4): 260-271. DOI: 10.1136/oem.17.4.260

[4] Britton M. The epidemiology of mesothelioma. Seminars in Oncology. 2002;**29**(1):18-25. DOI: 10.1053/ sonc.2002.30237

[5] Agudo A, González CA, Bleda MJ, et al. Occupation and risk of malignant pleural mesothelioma: A case–control study in Spain. American Journal of Industrial Medicine. 2000;**37**(2): 159-168. DOI: 10.1002/(SICI)1097-0274(200002)37:2<159: AID-AJIM1>3.0.CO;2-0

[6] Magnani C, Agudo A, González CA, et al. Multicentric study on malignant pleural mesothelioma and non-occupational exposure to asbestos. British Journal of Cancer. 2000;**83**(1):104. DOI: 10.1054/ bjoc.2000.1161

[7] Rödelsperger K, Jöckel K-H, Pohlabeln H, Römer W, Woitowitz H-J. Asbestos and man-made vitreous fibers as risk factors for diffuse malignant mesothelioma: Results from a German hospital-based case-control study. American Journal of Industrial Medicine. 2001;**39**(3):262-275. DOI: 10.1002/1097-0274(200103)39:3<262:: AID-AJIM1014>3.0.CO;2-R

[8] Lacourt A, Gramond C, Rolland P, et al. Occupational and non-occupational attributable risk of asbestos exposure for malignant pleural mesothelioma. Thorax. 2014;**69**(6):532-539. DOI: 10.1136/ thoraxjnl-2013-203744

[9] Markowitz S. Asbestos-related lung cancer and malignant mesothelioma of the pleura: Selected current issues. Seminars in Respiratory and Critical Care Medicine. 2015;**36**(03):334-346. DOI: 10.1055/s-0035-1549449

[10] Maxim LD, Niebo R, Utell MJ. Are pleural plaques an appropriate endpoint for risk analyses? Inhalation Toxicology. 2015;**27**:321-334

[11] Pairon JC, Laurent F, Rinaldo M, Clin B, Andujar P, et al. Pleural plaque and the risk of pleural mesothelioma. Journal of the National Cancer Institute. 2013;**105**:293-301

[12] Hourihane D, Lessof L, Richardson P. Hyaline and calcified pleural plaques as an index of exposure to asbestos. A study of radiological and pathological features of 100 cases with a consideration of epidemiology. British Medical Journal. 1966;**1**:1069-1074

[13] Doll R. Mortality from lung cancer in asbestos workers. British Journal of Industrial Medicine. 1955;**12**(2):81-86

[14] Roggli VI, Sharma A, Butnor KJ, Sporn T, Vollmer RT. Malignant mesothelioma and occupational exposure to asbestos: A clinicopathological correlation of 1445 cases. Ultrastructural Pathology. 2002;**26**:55-65

[15] Marinaccio A, Corfiati M, Binazzi A, et al. The epidemiology of malignant mesotheliomas in women: gender differences and modalities of asbestos exposure. Occupational

and Environmental Medicine. 2017;**75**(4):254-262

[16] Lemen RA. Mesothelioma from asbestos exposures: Epidemiologic patterns and impact in the United States. Journal of Toxicology & Environmental Health Part B: Critical Reviews. 2016;**19**:250-265

[17] Dawson A, Gibbs AR, Pooley FD, Griffiths DM, Hoy J. Malignant mesothelioma in in women. Thorax. 1993;**48**:269-274

[18] Tukiainen P, nickels J, Taskinen E, Nyberg M. Pulmonary granulomatous reaction: talc pneumoconiosis or chronic sarcoidosis? British Journal of Industrial Medicine. 1984;**41**:84-87

[19] Noppen M. Talc pleurodesis, Uptodate. Wolters Kluwer. 2019. pp. 1-17

[20] Stuart BO. Deposition and clearance of inhaled particles. Environmental Health Perspectives. 1976;**16**:41-53

[21] Bethune N. Pleural podrage: New technique for the deliberate production of pleural adhesion as preliminary to lobectomy. The Journal of Thoracic Surgery. 1935;**4**:251

[22] Rossi VF, Vargas FS, Marchi E, et al. Acute inflammatory response secondary to intrapleural administration of two types of talc. The European Respiratory Journal. 2010;**35**:396-401

[23] Genofre EH, Marchi E, Vargas FS. Inflammation and clinical repercussions of pleurodesis induced by intropleural talc administration. Clinics. 2007;**62**:627

[24] Aust AE, Eveleigh JF. Mechanaisms of DNA oxidation. Proceedings of the Society for Experimental Biology and Medicine. 1999;**222**:246-252

[25] Katsnelson BA, Mokronosova KA. Non-fibrous mineral dust and malignant tumors. An epidemiologic study of mortality. Journal of Occupational Medicine. 1979;**21**:15-20

[26] Beck B, Konetzke GW, Sturm W. Asbestos and mesothelioma in GDR. Archivum Immunologiae et Therapiae Experimentalis. 1982;**30**:229-233

[27] Werner I. Zur anwsenheit von asbest in talkproben. Atemschutz informationen. 1982;**21**:5-7

[28] Gordon RE, Fitzgerald S, Millette JR. Asbestos in commercial talc cosmetic talcum powder as a cause of mesothelioma in women. International Journal of Occupational and Environmental Health. 2014;**20**:318-332

[29] Muller WF, Schmadicke E, Okrusch M, Schussler U. Intergrowths between anthophyllite, gedrite, calcic amphibole, cummingtonite, talc and chlorite in a metamorphosed ultrmafic rock of the KTB ilot hole, Bavaria. European Journal of Mineralogy. 2003;**15**:295-307

[30] Cramer DW, Welch WR, Scully RE, Wojciechowski CA. Ovarian cancer and talc: A case-control study. Cancer. 1982;**50**:372-376

[31] Cramer DW, Liberman RF, Titus-Ernstoff L, Welch WR, Greenberg ER, Baron JA, et al. Genital talc exposure and the risk of ovarian cancer. International Journal of Cancer. 1999;**81**:351-356

[32] Larson D, Powers A, Ambrosi J-P, et al. Investigating palygorskite's role in the development of mesotheliom in southern Nevada: Insites into fiber-induced carcinogenicity. Journal of Toxicology & Environmental Health Part B: Critical Reviews. 2016;**19**:213-230

Chapter 4

Bronchopleural Fistula: Causes, Diagnoses and Management

Güntuğ Batıhan and Kenan Can Ceylan

Abstract

Bronchopleural fistula (BPF) is a pathological communication between the bronchial tree and pleural space. This clinical condition, which has high mortality and morbidity, is one of the major therapeutic challenges for clinicians even today. BPF may result from a lung neoplasm, necrotizing pneumonia, empyema, blunt and penetrating lung injuries, and a complication of surgical procedures. Lung resection is the most common cause of BPF, and this chapter will focus more on this topic. Frequency ranges from 4.5 to 20% after pneumonectomy and from 0.5 to 1% after lobectomy. Several risk factors have been defined in the development of postoperative BPF; preoperative radiotherapy, pulmonary infection, diabetes, right pneumonectomy, a long bronchial stump, residual cancer at the stump (R1 and R2 resection), and the need for postoperative ventilation (especially with high PEEP). BPFs are divided, based on the time elapsed since surgery, into early or late fistula. This grouping is important in management of patient treatment. In early BPF, surgical treatment is generally the preferred treatment modality, whereas in late BPF, conservative approach is preferred. The management of BPF is still one of the most complex challenges encountered by the thoracic surgeons; so prevention is the best way to manage postoperative BPF.

Keywords: bronchopleural fistula, complication, lung resection, empyema

1. Introduction

Bronchopleural fistula (BPF) has been defined as a direct communication between the bronchus and pleural cavity. Some authors have grouped BPFs as central and peripheral according to their locations [1]. While a central BPF defines connection between pleura and tracheobronchial three, a peripheral BPF defines connection between the pleura and airway distal to segmental bronchi or lung parenchyma. In literature, the term of "alveolopleural fistula" is also used to describe peripheral BPFs.

Nonsurgical conditions like trauma, chronic necrotizing pneumonia, empyema, radiotherapy, bulla, or cyst rupture can cause BPF, but the most common cause is lung resection. Frequency ranges from 4.5 to 20% after pneumonectomy and from 0.5 to 1% after lobectomy. BPF-related mortality ranges from 18 to 71% in the literature [2–4]. Because of high morbidity and mortality rates, it is important to define risk factors and apply preventative methods especially in groups of risky patients.

Many authors have divided postoperative BPFs into two groups according to time of onset. There is no consensus about these definitions in the literature, but generally, early BPF was defined as fistula occurring within 30 days after the initial operation. Late BPF was defined as fistulas occurring after more than 30 days. It is established that early BPFs are most commonly associated with a failure in surgical technique and mostly, it can be repaired with reoperation [1, 3, 5].

Late BPFs are typically secondary to patient-related factors and almost always coexist with empyema, and it usually required complex, long-term, and exhausting treatment process for both the patient and the surgeon.

2. Risk factors

BPF is most commonly encountered after lung resections; therefore, establishing risk factors is important to prevent patients from this highly mortal complication.

Numerous risk factors have been associated with BPF development in the literature [3–6]. We divided these risk factors into three groups: patient-related factors, surgeon-related factors, and anatomic factors.

Age (>60), gender (male), neoadjuvant radiation therapy, diabetes mellitus, malnutrition, smoking, chronic steroid/immunosuppressive usage, and need for postoperative mechanic ventilation can be classified as a patient-related risk factor. Induction chemotherapy has been cited as a risk factor for postpneumonectomy BPF but there is not any increased risk for bronchoplastic procedures.

A large number of studies have reported an increased risk for BPF due to postoperative mechanical ventilation usage after pneumonectomy. Therefore, to prevent bronchial stump from barotrauma extubation must be achieved at the earliest time after surgery.

A low forced expiratory volume in 1 second and low carbon monoxide diffusing capacity were also defined as risk factors for postoperative BPF occurrence.

Besides these patient-related risk factors, several anatomic disadvantages were defined for right-sided pneumonectomy:

i. According to cadaveric studies, presence of two left-sided and one right-sided bronchial artery supply is the most common configuration.

ii. While the left main bronchus is protected under the aortic arch and surrounded by mediastinal tissue, the right bronchial stump has no such coverage.

iii. The right main bronchus is wider, and more vertical than the left main bronchus. This condition facilitates secretion retention on the right main bronchial stump.

Early BPFs are usually related with technical failure during surgery. The most common causes of this condition are poorly secured knots, stapler misfiring, and high anastomotic tension. Other surgeon-related risk factors are extensive mediastinal lymphadenectomy and peribronchial dissection, long bronchial stump and not coverage the bronchial stump with viable tissue.

3. Clinical presentations and diagnosis

The size and the time of occurrence of the BPF are major determinants of the clinical presentation but, patients often have infection-related symptoms like: fever, cough with serosanguinous or purulent sputum, night sweats, and chills.

Expectoration and respiratory symptoms typically worsen with the patient lying on the side opposite to the one involving the fistula. Flooding of the infected contents of the pleural space to the contralateral lung can lead to severe pneumonia or respiratory distress syndrome.

If the patient has a chest tube massive and prolonged air leakage would be an important clinical clue for BPF.

White blood cell count and systemic inflammation markers are often elevated.

Chest radiogram often revealed a decrease in the fluid level and enlargement in the ipsilateral pleural cavity. Due to the contamination of the contralateral lung by the infected content of the pleural cavity, parenchymal infiltration can be seen.

Computed tomography of the chest can depict mediastinal emphysema, parenchymal infiltration, and enlargement of the pleural cavity, but its success at demonstrating the presence of the BPF is controversial. By the imaging of the continuation of a bronchus or the lung parenchyma to the pleural space, definitive diagnosis of the fistula can be made (**Figures 1** and **2**). Westcott et al. reported sensitivity of the chest CT as 50% at demonstrating the presence of the peripheral BPFs. Seo et al. reported that chest CT succeed to demonstrate direct or indirect signs of BPF 86% of the patients with central, and 100% of the patients with peripheral BPFs [7, 8].

In the presence of clinical or radiological suspicion of BPF, bronchoscopy must be applied to examine the bronchial stump. Presence of pleural fluid leakage or/and air bubbling in the bronchial stump is pathognomonic (**Figures 3** and **4**).

Reconstruction of 2-dimensional, helical CT images provides noninvasive intraluminal evaluation of the bronchus named as "virtual bronchoscopy" [9]. This technique can provide additional benefits, especially, planning endobronchial instrumentation, but it is not an essential diagnostic method of fistula.

Less frequently ^{133}xenon or ^{99}technetium ventilation scintigraphy can be used to identify BPF by visualization of the radioactive isotopes in the empty pleural cavity. Mark et al. used ^{99}technetium ventilation scintigraphy in 28 postpneumonectomy patients for the detection of BPF and reported sensitivity of 78% and a specificity of 100% [10, 11]. Although, this is a noninvasive diagnostic procedure, it is not practical and easy-to-use, and has no additional benefit to the detection of underlying lung disease.

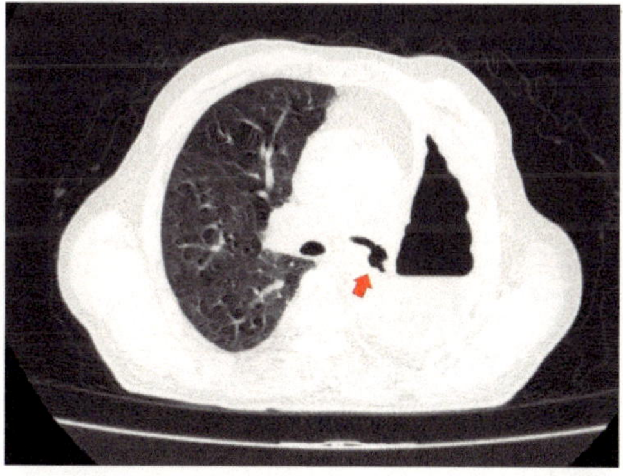

Figure 1.
Left sided BPF is seen in the Chest CT. BPF may not always be as clear as this CT image.

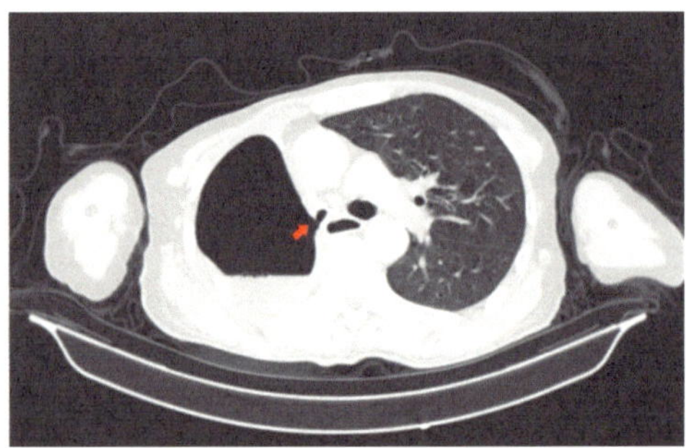

Figure 2.
Another chest CT image shows right sided BPF. Chest CT also allows the examination of the remaining lung for possible pneumonic infiltrations and metastases.

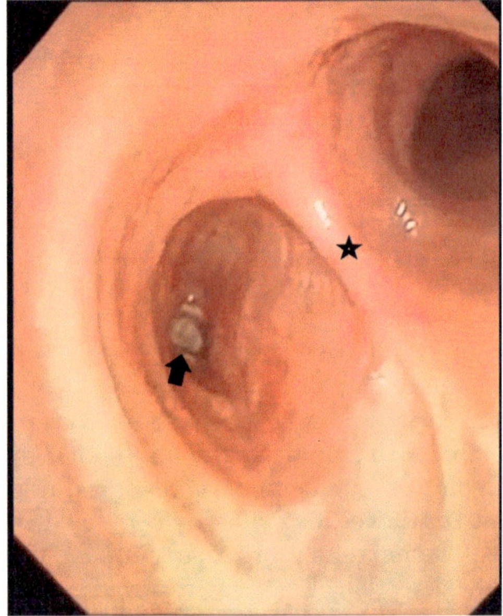

Figure 3.
Bronchoscope view of the left-sided BPF (arrow) (Asterix shows the main carina). In bronchoscopy, the fistula patency may not always be clearly seen. Air bubbles originating from the stump of the bronchus may be the only sign of the BPF.

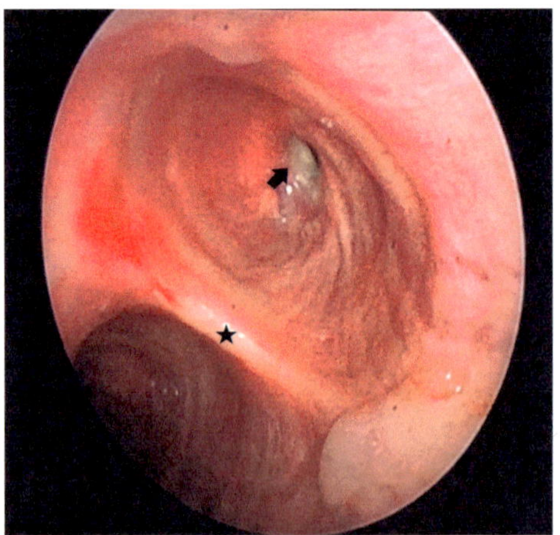

Figure 4.
Bronchoscope view of the right-sided BPF (arrow) (Asterix shows the main carina).

4. Management

The management of the BPF needs prolonged hospitalization, complex surgical procedures, and close follow-up, but first step in the treatment is management of the life-threatening conditions like sepsis, tension pneumothorax, and respiratory failure. Protection of the contralateral lung from aspiration of the pleural fluid is important to reduce the risk of pneumonia and respiratory failure. Therefore, chest tube must be applied to ensure the drainage of the pleural cavity. Broad spectrum antibiotic therapy against Gram-Positive, Gram-Negative, and anaerobic microorganisms must be initiated, and it should be tailored based on the results of culture-antibiograms.

Early BPFs are mostly associated with failure in the surgical technique. Repairment of the bronchial stump with re-operation is the best treatment modality in these patients.

Patients with late BPF mostly have poor medical condition and major surgical approaches cannot be applied. Conservative treatment modalities like drainage and reduction of the pleural space, pleural irrigation, antibiotics, and nutritional supplementation. Boudaya et al. reported their experience with conservative management of postresectional BPF in 17 patients and BPF is successfully closed in 16 patients [12].

Various endoscopic techniques for the control of small BPFs have been reported, especially in patients with poor condition. Sealants, fibrin glue, coils, and endobronchial silicon or metal stents have been used to treat small BPFs (ranging from 0.8 to 1.0 mm). Dutau et al. used self-expanding metal stents in seven patients with large fistulas (>6 mm) and reported improvement in patients' respiratory parameters in early postoperative period [13].

4.1 Surgical interventions for infection control

Besides conservative treatments, several surgical procedures to treat BPFs have been defined in the literature. Main objectives in these surgical interventions are debridement of the pleural space, minimizing the residual pleural cavity, closure of the fistula, and reinforcement of the bronchial stump with autologous tissue.

There are several factors in choosing the appropriate surgical method:

1. Medical condition of the patient

2. Time of onset of the fistula

3. Size and localization of the fistula

4. State of the pleural cavity

4.1.1 Video-assisted thoracoscopic surgery (VATS)

In the presence of pleural infection together with the fistula, tube-thoracostomy must be applied in all cases. Pleural irrigation with antibiotic and povidone-iodine solutions is suggested in sterilization of the infected postpneumonectomy pleural cavity but this treatment modality alone cannot provide sufficient debridement, especially in patients with late fistulas and cause prolong hospitalization.

VATS is a useful method to obtain drainage and debridement of the infected pleural cavity. Single port is usually sufficient in most cases; material and debris can be safely removed with surgical instruments and in the presence of small BPFs (<3 mm) fibrine glue can be applied. Hollaus et al. applied videothoracoscopic debridement in nine patients and defined it as an efficient method to treat postpneumonectomy empyema [14]. Gossot et al. reported series of 11 patients with postpneumonectomy empyema. These 11 patients underwent videothoracoscopic debridement and 8 of 11 patients discharged without need of additional surgical procedures [15]. These similar studies have shown that VATS is a feasible option for treatment in select patients with PPE and small BPF.

4.1.2 Open window thoracostomy

In the presence of empyema drainage of the pleural cavity is essential to control the septic status of the patient. Different kinds of drainage techniques were defined in the literature. Open-window thoracostomy was first described by Robinson in 1916 in patients with nontuberculous empyema and Eloesser has revised this procedure for patients with tuberculous empyema [16, 17]. This procedure contains:

1. Segmental resection of 2–3 ribs

2. Creation of a skin flap (Muscle should be preserved if possible)

3. Marsupialization of the cavity

With this procedure, epithelialized thoracostomy window is obtained and effective drainage is ensured.

After this operation, the wound is packed at least daily with gauze moistened with normal saline. Granulation tissue in the wound begins to form over time and when the pleural space is clean closure of the window can be considered.

It is very important to have a good cooperation with patient and relatives for this treatment modality and they should be informed that this treatment procedure may require several weeks.

4.1.3 Clagett procedure

Clagett and Geraci described a two-step treatment technique for the management of postpneumonectomy empyema in 1963 [18]. Step 1 contains the open window thoracostomy to drain the septic cavity. Step 2 contains obliteration of the pleural cavity with antibiotic solution. Pairolero and Arnold has modified this procedure and described transposition of a well-vascularized extrathoracic muscle as an intermediate step [19]. With this modification, further reinforcement of the bronchial stump was ensured.

Clagett procedure shows a success rate (OWT closed without PPE recurrence) of 61–89% with a mortality rate between 0 and 24% in the literature.

4.2 Surgically closure of a bronchopleural fistula

Large BPF can cause loss in the tidal volume, aspiration of infected pleural fluid, and respiratory distress. Therefore, bronchial defect must be controlled, especially in patients with large fistulas, for this purpose, two major approaches were defined in the literature.

4.2.1 Transpleural approach

Transpleural approach is the most common method to closure of the BPF (**Figure 5**). First, BPF must be identified. By careful dissection, bronchus must be mobilized as close to the carina as possible to provide adequate length. Aggressive

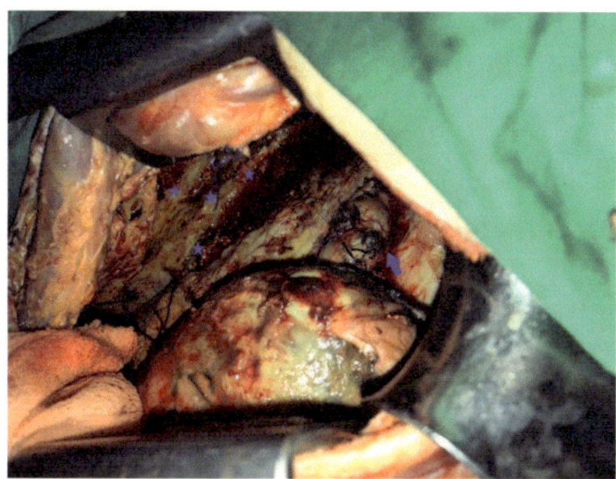

Figure 5.
Image of the left thoracic cavity of the patient with BPF and empyema. Pleural debris and plaques covering the chest wall are seen (Asterix). Infected vascular stumps also are seen (arrow).

dissection and devascularization of the proximal bronchus should be avoided because of the risk of failure of the repair and recurrence of BPF. Stapler devices can be used if there is a sufficient length in the bronchial stump. Manual suturation also can be applied above the BPF. After repairment, bronchial stump must be buttressed with well-vascularized tissue such as extrathoracic muscle, omentum, or diaphragm flap.

4.2.2 Transsternal transpericardial approach

In some cases, surgical management of BPF may be challenging through a lateral transpleural approach. Presence of short bronchial stumps, left-sided BPF, necrotic bronchial stumps and/or history of prior BPF closures via thoracotomy are the main reasons that make transpleural approach difficult. In these cases, transsternal transpericardial approach would be a good alternative to transpleural approach [20, 21]. This approach provides work in healthy, inflammation-free planes. Therefore, in this technique, isolation of the airway is easier and safer than others. Biggest benefit of this technique is that it provides the opportunity to work in a healthy plane. Retraction of the superior vena cava and aorta laterally provide sufficient exposure to make a successful repairment. It is also possible to achieve transpericardial approach by anterior thoracic incision with division of multiple costal cartilages which was described by Padhi and Lynn [22]. This approach was found to be a difficult and complicated compared to transsternal approach. Therefore, transsternal transpericardial approach has become more widely used among surgeons in the repairment of BPF.

4.2.3 Thoracoplasty

One of the major concerns in the treatment of the BPF is obliteration of the persistent space after control of pleural infection. Thoracoplasty is originally considered as a treatment for active tuberculosis but this procedure is also functional for obliterate pleural space with the viable tissue of the chest wall in the cases of BPF. This is achieved by resection of multiple ribs. Traditional thoracoplasty requires removal of the first 11 ribs periosteum, and intercostal muscles with associated neurovascular bundles. After removal of these structures, skin and thoracic muscles fill the pleural cavity. As can be expected, this procedure has high mortality and morbidity rates and is now abandoned. Removing fewer than five ribs named as "tailored" thoracoplasty is still in use especially in the treatment of chronic BPFs [23, 24].

It would be rational to use these treatment modalities in combination to deal with space problem. Tailored thoracoplasty, muscle transposition, omentoplasty, and diaphragm flabs can be used and combined with each other. Clinical condition and performance status of the patient are also important for selection of the best method in the treatment of BPF.

5. Bronchoscopic management of BPF

Various endoscopic techniques like bronchoscopic application of sealants, fibrin glue, silver nitrate cautery, coils, and endobronchial stents for the control of small BPFs have been reported [25–29]. There is no consensus on which method is most effective for BPF closure. We use endoscopic techniques only for the patients with poor clinical condition and not for proper major surgical intervention. Proper technique must be selected depending on the length of the bronchial stump, the location, and size of the fistula (**Figures 6** and 7).

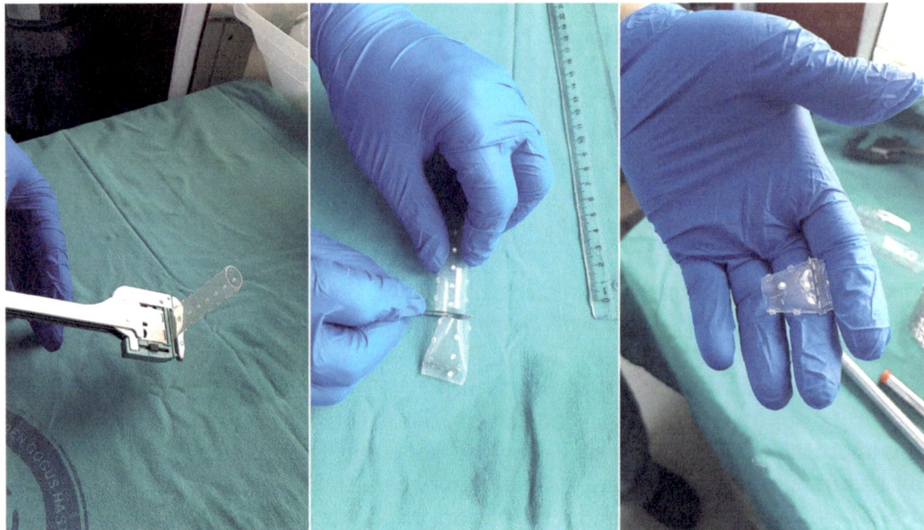

Figure 6.
Image of the customized (closed in one side with a stapler) silicone stent.

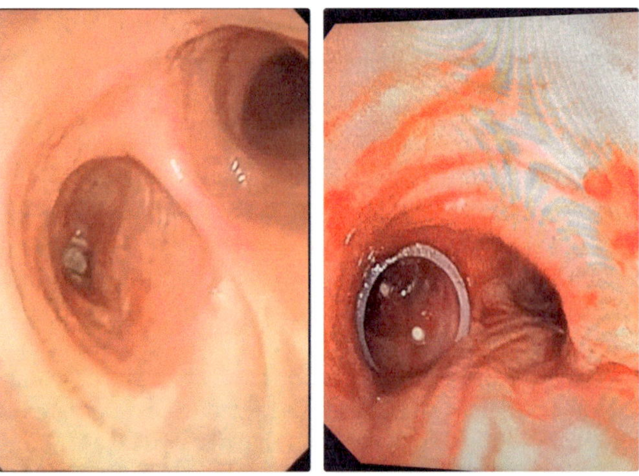

Figure 7.
Left-sided BPF was closed with customized silicone stent. After this procedure, air drainage from the chest tube was decreased and respiratory condition of the patient was improved.

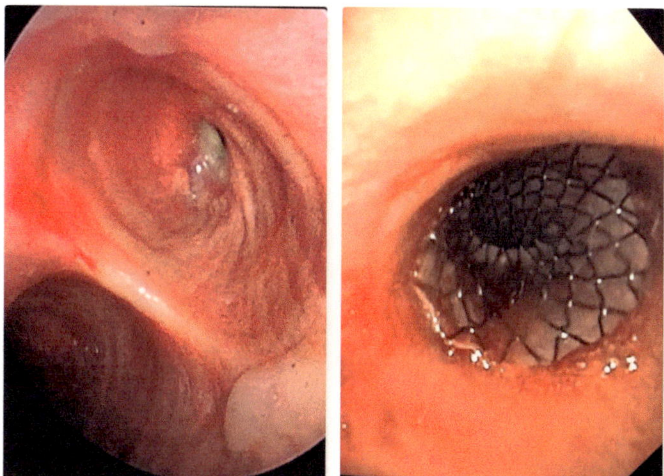

Figure 8.
Bronchoscope image of the right-sided BPF. It was closed with self-expandable metallic stent.

We often prefer metallic J-stents and silicon Y-stents (**Figure 8**). The most seen complication of these stents is migration and occlusion with secretion. Migration and occlusion of the stent can cause severe respiratory distress. Retention of the secretion can also cause contamination of the remaining lung and resulted in severe pneumonia.

Despite these complications, in selected patients, endobronchial stents can reduce air leakage and prevent remaining lung from contamination with pleural fluid.

6. Prevention of bronchopleural fistula in pulmonary resection-bronchial stump coverage

To prevent postpneumonectomy bronchopleural fistula, coverage of the bronchial stump is recommended, especially for patients with high risk of BPF.

Pedicled intercostal and extrathoracic muscles, diaphragm, pericardium, pericardial fat pad, and pleura can be used to make a flap to coverage the bronchial stump [30–32]. There is no consensus for best bronchial stump coverage method and related techniques with several complications were defined in the literature.

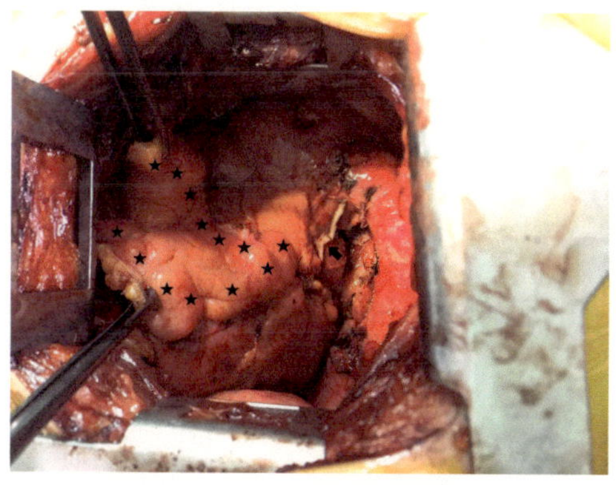

Figure 9.
Pericardial fat pad (Asterix) is very useful material to coverage of the bronchial stump. It is dissected from surrounding tissues by preserving the vascular pedicle. Once the fat pad has been mobilized, it is then rotated over the hilum to cover the bronchial staple line (arrows).

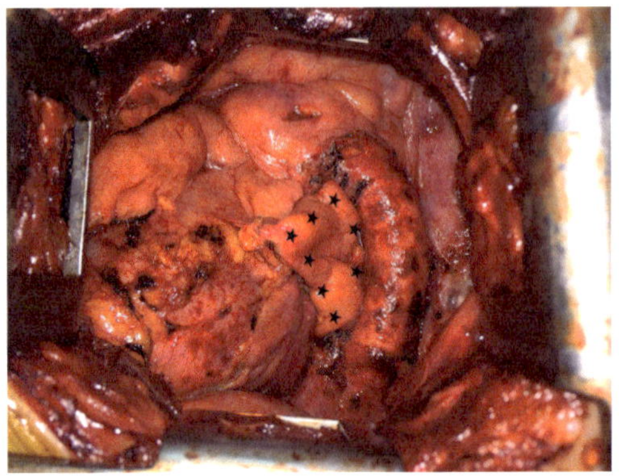

Figure 10.
The view of the thoracic cavity after coverage of the left main bronchial stump.

Diaphragm flaps can cause visceral herniation. The pedicled intercostal muscle flap is useful method for coverage of the bronchial stump but developing heterotopic ossification can cause severe problems. Omentum is a great tissue to promote re-vascularization and healing of the bronchial stump but it requires the opening of the abdominal cavity [33]. Pericardial fat pad coverage appears to be safe and feasible when compared with other coverage techniques (**Figures 9** and **10**). It can be applied without risk of additional comorbidity and composes a mechanical barrier between bronchial stump and pleural cavity.

7. Conclusion

In modern thoracic surgery, bronchopleural fistula is still associated with significant morbidity and mortality. Treatment techniques have evolved and there are many options to use in patients with BPF, therefore surgeon must evaluate clinical status of the patient, the size, and location of the BPF and the status of the pleural cavity to select the treatment method that will show the most benefit.

It is important to remember that the best treatment is to prevent the disease. Therefore, rigorous surgical technique and bronchial stump coverage are the main steps in the treatment.

Conflict of interest

The authors declare no conflict of interest.

Appendices and nomenclature

BPF	bronchopleural fistula
CT	computed tomography
VATS	video-assisted thoracoscopic surgery

Author details

Güntuğ Batıhan* and Kenan Can Ceylan
Department of Thoracic Surgery, Dr Suat Seren Chest Diseases and Surgery Medical Practice and Research Center, University of Health Sciences, Izmir, Turkey

*Address all correspondence to: gbatihan@hotmail.com

IntechOpen

© 2019 The Author(s). Licensee IntechOpen. This chapter is distributed under the terms of the Creative Commons Attribution License (http://creativecommons.org/licenses/by/3.0), which permits unrestricted use, distribution, and reproduction in any medium, provided the original work is properly cited. CC BY

References

[1] Okuda M, Go T, Yokomise H. Risk factor of bronchopleural fistula after general thoracic surgery: Review article. General Thoracic and Cardiovascular Surgery. Dec 2017;**65**(12):679-685. DOI: 10.1007/s11748-017-0846-1. [Epub 2017 Oct 12]

[2] Deschamps C, Bernard A, Nichols FC 3rd, et al. Empyema and bronchopleural fistula after pneumonectomy: Factors affecting incidence. The Annals of Thoracic Surgery. 2001;**72**:243-247 [discussion: 248]

[3] Pforr A, Pages PB, Baste JM, et al. A predictive score for bronchopleural fistula established using the French database EPITHOR. The Annals of Thoracic Surgery. 2016;**101**:287-293

[4] Wright CD, Wain JC, Mathisen DJ, et al. Postpneumonectomy bronchopleural fistula after sutured bronchial closure: Incidence, risk factors, and management. The Journal of Thoracic and Cardiovascular Surgery. 1996;**112**:1367-1371

[5] Asamura H, Naruke T, Tsuchiya R, et al. Bronchopleural fistulas associated with lung cancer operations. Univariate and multivariate analysis of risk factors, management, and outcome. The Journal of Thoracic and Cardiovascular Surgery. 1992;**104**:1456-1464

[6] Martin J, Ginsberg RJ, Abolhoda A, et al. Morbidity and mortality after neoadjuvant therapy for lung cancer: The risks of right pneumonectomy. The Annals of Thoracic Surgery. 2001;**72**:1149-1154

[7] Wescott JL, Volpe JP. Peripheral bronchopleural fistula: CT evaluation in 20 patients with pneumonia, emphyema, or postoperative air leak. Radiology. 1995;**196**:175-181

[8] Seo H, Kim TJ, Jin KN, Lee KW. Multi-detector row computed tomography evaluation of bronchopleural fistula: Correlation with clinical, bronchoscopic, and surgical findings. Journal of Computer Assisted Tomography. 2010;**34**:13-18

[9] Gaur P, Dunne R, Colson Y, Gill R. Bronchopleural fistula and the role of contemporary imaging. The Journal of Thoracic and Cardiovascular Surgery. 2013;**148**. DOI: 10.1016/j.jtcvs.2013.11.009

[10] Nielsen KR, Blake LM, Mark JB, DeCampli W, McDougall IR. Localization of bronchopleural fistula using ventilation scintigraphy. Journal of Nuclear Medicine. 1994;**35**:867-869

[11] Raja S, Rice TW, Neumann DR, Saha GB, Khandekar S, MacIntyre WJ, et al. Scintigraphic detection of post-pneumonectomy bronchopleural fistulae. European Journal of Nuclear Medi^c^ine. 1999;**26**:215-219

[12] Boudaya MS, Smadhi H, Zribi H, et al. Conservative management of postoperative bronchopleural fistulas. The Journal of Thoracic and Cardiovascular Surgery. 2013;**146**:575-579

[13] Dutau H, Breen DP, Gomez C, et al. The integrated place of tracheobronchial stents in the multidisciplinary management of large post-pneumonectomy fistulas: Our experience using a novel customised conical self-expandable metallic stent. European Journal of Cardio-Thoracic Surgery. 2011;**39**:185-189. DOI: 10.1016/j.ejcts.2010.05.020

[14] Hollaus PH, Lax F, Wurnig PN, et al. Videothoracoscopic debridement of the postpneumonectomy space in empyema. The European Journal

of Cardio-Thoracic Surgery. 1999;**16**:283-286

[15] Gossot D, Stern JB, Galetta D, et al. Thoracoscopic management of postpneumonectomy empyema. The Annals of Thoracic Surgery. 2004;**78**:273-276

[16] Robinson S. The treatment of chronic non-tuberculous empyema. Surgery, Gynecology & Obstetrics. 1916;**64**

[17] Eloesser L. An operation for tuberculous empyema. Surgery, Gynecology & Obstetrics. 1935;**60**:1096-1097

[18] Clagett OT, Geraci JE. A procedure for the management of postpneumonectomy empyema. The Journal of Thoracic and Cardiovascular Surgery. 1963;**45**:141-145

[19] Pairolero PC, Arnold PG, Trastek VF, et al. Postpneumonectomy empyema. The role of intrathoracic muscle transposition. The Journal of Thoracic and Cardiovascular Surgery. 1990;**99**:958-966 [discussion: 966-8]

[20] Deschamps C, Allen MS, Miller DL, et al. Management of postpneumonectomy empyema and bronchopleural fistula. Seminars in Thoracic and Cardiovascular Surgery. 2001;**13**:13-19

[21] Abruzzini P. Trattamento chirurgico delle fistole del bronco principale consecutive a pneumonectomia per tubercolosi. Chirur Torac. 1961;**14**:165-171

[22] Padhi RK, Lynn RB. The management of bronchopleural fistulas. The Journal of Thoracic and Cardiovascular Surgery. 1960;**39**:385-393

[23] Goldstraw P. Treatment of postpneumonectomy empyema: The case for fenestration. Thorax. 1979;**34**:740-745

[24] Estlander JA. Sur le resection des cotes dans l'empyeme chronique. The Medico-Chirurgical Review. 1891;**8**:885-888

[25] Lois M, Noppen M. Bronchopleural fistulas: An overview of the problem with special focus on endoscopic management. Chest. 2005;**128**:3955-3965

[26] Jones NC, Kirk AJ, Edwards RD. Bronchopleural fistula treated with a covered wallstent. The Annals of Thoracic Surgery. 2006;**81**:364. DOI: 10.1016/j.athoracsur.2004.09.054

[27] Klotz LV, Gesierich W, Schott-Hildebrand S, et al. Endobronchial closure of bronchopleural fistula using Amplatzer device. Journal of Thoracic Disease. 2015;**7**:1478-1482

[28] Hamid UI, Jones JM. Closure of a bronchopleural fistula using glue. Interactive Cardiovascular and Thoracic Surgery. 2011;**13**:117-118. DOI: 10.1510/icvts.2011.270397

[29] Amaral B, Feijó S. Fistula of the stump: A novel approach with a "stapled" stent. Journal of Bronchology and Interventional Pulmonology. 2015;**22**:365-366. DOI: 10.1097/LBR.0000000000000172

[30] Klepetko W, Taghavi S, Pereszlenyi A, et al. Impact of different coverage techniques on incidence of postpneumonectomy stump fistula. European Journal of Cardio-Thoracic Surgery. 1999;**15**:758-763

[31] Anderson TM, Miller JI Jr. Use of pleura, azygos vein, pericardium, and muscle flaps in tracheobronchial surgery. The Annals of Thoracic Surgery. 1995;**60**:729-733

[32] Anderson TM, Miller JI Jr. Surgical technique and application of pericardial

fat pad and pericardiophrenic grafts. The Annals of Thoracic Surgery. 1995;**59**:1590-1591

[33] Okumura Y, Takeda S, Asada H, et al. Surgical results for chronic empyema using omental pedicled flap: Long-term follow-up study. The Annals of Thoracic Surgery. 2005;**79**:1857-1861. DOI: 10.1016/j.athoracsur.2005.01.001

Chapter 5

Solitary Fibrous Tumours of the Pleura

Alberto Sandri, Alessandro Maraschi, Matteo Gagliasso, Carlotta Cartia, Roberta Rapanà, Simona Sobrero, Federica Massa, Luisella Righi and Francesco Ardissone

Abstract

Solitary fibrous tumours of the pleura (SFTP) are rare neoplasms originating from one of the components of the sub-mesothelial connective layer underlying the pleura. They are the most common non-mesothelial primary pleural neoplasms but still remain relatively rare. Their behaviour is mostly indolent; however, some may de-differentiate into malignant and aggressive tumours. Surgical resection is the mainstay treatment for SFTP, even more so in case of voluminous masses, due to compression onto lung, mediastinum and great vessels. In this chapter, we discuss the disease characteristics reported in the literature with respect to clinical presentation, diagnosis and treatment; also, we will discuss the results of patients treated for SFTP who underwent a surgical treatment in our unit of thoracic surgery.

Keywords: solitary fibrous tumour of the pleura, pleura, surgery, resection, recurrence

1. Introduction

The pleura is composed of two sections: the mesothelium, a single layer of flattened cells, and a deeper sub-mesothelial layer formed by a matrix of collagen, elastic fibres, lymphatic and blood vessels.

Primary pleural tumours may originate from any of the pleural components.

Out of all the pleural neoplasms, 90% are malignant mesotheliomas, 5% are solitary fibrous pleural tumours (SFPT) and the remaining 5% consists of less frequent variants (**Table 1**) [1].

Solitary fibrous tumours of the pleura originate from one of the components of the sub-mesothelial connective layer; therefore, its origin is mesenchymal. It usually presents as a well-circumscribed mass of occasional finding at chest X-rays performed for other reasons, since it presents asymptomatically.

SFTPs are the most common non-mesothelial primary pleural neoplasms, but still remain relatively rare. In fact, to date, <2000 cases have been reported in the literature [2]. They originate most frequently from the visceral pleura and have a benign course; only in a small percentage of cases (10–15%) their behaviour is

Benign
Solitary fibrous tumour of the pleura
Calcifying fibrous tumour
Adenomatoid tumour
Sclerosing pneumocytoma (hemangioma)
Pleural lipoma
Pleural Schwannoma
Malign
Solitary fibrous tumour of the pleura
Desmoplastic small round cell tumour
Localized malignant mesothelioma
Primary pleural thymomas
Synovial sarcoma of the pleura
Primary pleural liposarcoma
Fibrosarcomas of the pleura and desmoid tumours
Vascular origin
Epithelioid hemangioendothelioma
Angiosarcoma
Epithelioid angiosarcoma
Lymphatic
Primary pleural lymphoma

Table 1.
Classification—rare pleural tumours.

malignant, presenting a de-differentiated pattern, aggressive clinical behaviour (invasion of adjacent organs or cardiac compression due to its huge mass) and a trend to relapse after several years, therefore requiring long-term follow-up.

Although surgery is the main approach to treating SFTPs, local and distant recurrences may be observed after a complete resection [3, 4].

In this chapter we will discuss the characteristics of the disease reported in the literature with respect to its clinical presentation, diagnosis and treatment; also, we will present the results of patients who underwent surgery for SFTP in our Department from 1989 to 2019.

2. Historical background

Lieutaud was the first to report a tumour of pleural origin in 1767 but the first report of what was thought to be a SFTP dates back to 1870 in the work of Wagner [5].

In 1931, Klemper and Rabin [6] provided the first pathological distinction for pleural tumours classifying them into diffuse and localised mesotheliomas. They assumed a sub-mesothelial mesenchymal origin for the localised type.

Eleven years later, Stout and Murray [7] described the typical histological feature of the fibrous tumour of the pleura, the so-called patternless pattern, initially thought to be a vascular neoplasm related to smooth muscle perivascular cells (pericytes), therefore naming it hemangiopericytoma.

Since its pathological features were first described, the nomenclature has become confused, and the disease has also been referred to as localised mesotheliomas, localised fibrous tumours, fibrous mesotheliomas, or pleural fibromas.

The introduction of electron microscope and immunohistochemistry clarified the hypothesis that SFTP does not originate from the mesothelial layer but from the sub-mesothelial, undifferentiated mesenchymal layer [8, 9].

SFTP is now recognised as occurring anywhere in the body, including soft tissue and viscera, albeit with a peculiar predilection for body cavity sites, including pleura, peritoneum, and meninges.

In recent studies, SFTPs distribution is as follows: 30% in the thoracic cavity (pleura, lungs and mediastinum); 30% in the peritoneal cavity, in the retroperitoneum or pelvis. When SFTP arise in the abdominal cavity it is mainly localised in the retroperitoneum followed by the pelvic soft tissue [10].

Nearly 20% of SFTPs are found in the head-neck district (including meninges). The remaining diseases develop in soft tissue of the trunk and extremities [11].

Data on presentation, clinical features and natural history of SFTPs are almost exclusively derived from retrospective series and case reports.

Since the discovery of SFTP, there has been some confusion in the classification by body site (pleural vs. extra-pleural), the histology (SFTP vs. hemangiopericytoma) and changes in diagnostic terminology has resulted in a fragmented and unsystematic approach to this uncommon neoplasm.

Robinson and Chmielecki's [12, 13] recent discovery of a common driver mutation for pleural and extra-thoracic SFTPs in 2013 drastically changed our understanding of SFTP pathogenesis and led to new opportunities for diagnosis, characterisation and treatment.

2.1 Clinical features

Usually, the SFTP is discovered in asymptomatic middle-aged adults (occasionally in children) and affects men and women equally. It is more common in the fifth and sixth decades of life. Some authors have reported that the tumour shows a slight predilection for women [2, 4, 14, 15].

It seems not to be associated with exposure to asbestos fibres exposure or tobacco smoke [16, 17].

Although the majority of SFTP are benign, it is reported that nearly 10–20% are malignant or show a malignant behaviour [18, 19].

Histologically, malignant tumours are classified according to England et al. [18] criteria:

- mitotic count with more than four mitosis/10 high power fields (HPF) (×400)
- presence of necrosis
- hyper cellularity as judged by nuclear crowding and overlapping
- presence of nuclear atypia

Mostly, patients are asymptomatic, but when they present symptoms, these usually include cough, chest pain, dyspnoea due to pleural effusion or the mass effect of the tumour. Haemoptysis and obstructive pneumonia may be observed as a result of airway obstruction. Chest pain has been reported more commonly with tumours arising from the parietal pleura.

A higher incidence of symptoms is also described in malignant variants [20], with a large variability of presentation varying from 43 to 73% [2, 14]; only few cases have been reported associated to paraneoplastic syndromes: 3% with hypertrophic pulmonary osteoarthropathy (HPO) and 2% with Doege-Potter syndrome [2].

2.2 Paraneoplastic syndromes

2.2.1 Hypertrophic pulmonary osteoarthropathy or Pierre Marie-Bamberger syndrome

Hypertrophic pulmonary osteoarthropathy (HPO) describes a rheumatoid like disease of the bones and joints. The symptoms include clubbing of the fingers and toes, stiffness of the joints, oedema over the ankles and occasionally the hands, arthralgia, and pain along the surfaces of the long bones, especially the tibia [20].

Finger pressure on the surface of the tibia can elicit pain before the onset of any radiographic evidence of SFTP.

When clubbing and HPO are attributed to a paraneoplastic syndrome, this is referred to as the Pierre Marie-Bamberger syndrome since they first described the symptoms in 1890 [21, 22].

This is reported in up to 20% of patients and it is more commonly associated with large tumours (>7 cm) [20].

Some authors have reported that these clinical features usually resolve within 2–5 months (or sometimes longer) after radical surgery and may reappear if the tumour relapses [3, 15, 18].

It is believed that local production of growth factors including PDGF and VEGF is implicated in the pathophysiology of HPO. In support of this, in a recent study the administration of zoledronate resulted in bone pain remission [23].

In another study, Hojo et al. suggested the abnormal production of hepatocyte growth factor as responsible for digital clubbing [24].

2.2.2 Hypoglycaemia (Doege-Potter syndrome)

The association between hypoglycaemia and a mesenchymal tumour has been reported for the first time in 1930 by Doege and Potter. This is present in <5% of patients affected by SFTP [25, 26].

Hypoglycaemia is equally distributed between benign and malignant SFTs albeit it occurs mostly in large peritoneal/pleural tumours [27].

Symptoms of hypoglycaemia include convulsions, syncope and coma and potentially death resulting from severe hypoglycaemia, if not corrected promptly.

Hypoglycaemia seems to be caused by an excessive production and secretion of a partially processed, high molecular weight form of insulin-like growth factor 2 (IGF-2) by the tumour [28]. The aberrant production of IGF-2 by the neoplasm is also the cause of refractory hypoglycaemia suppressing compensatory mechanism as gluconeogenesis in the liver and lipolysis in adipose tissue.

The paraneoplastic syndrome is generally cured after tumour's resection, with the return to normal levels of insulin within a few days after the operation [29].

2.3 Radiographic features

2.3.1 Chest X-ray

Generally, SFTPs are an occasional finding in chest X-ray performed for other reasons.

They appear as a solid, sharply marginated, well-circumscribed solitary lesion originating from the periphery of the chest or from a lung fissure. It may grow to remarkable dimensions, at times occupying the entirety of the hemithorax. It is very difficult, if not impossible, to distinguish them from other masses of the lung by means of a plain chest X-ray (**Figure 1**).

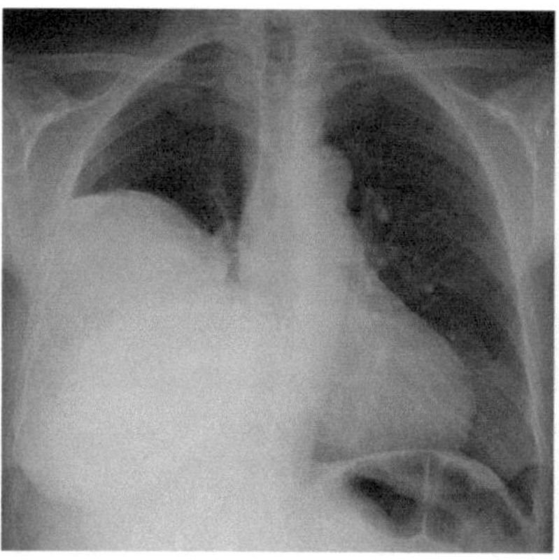 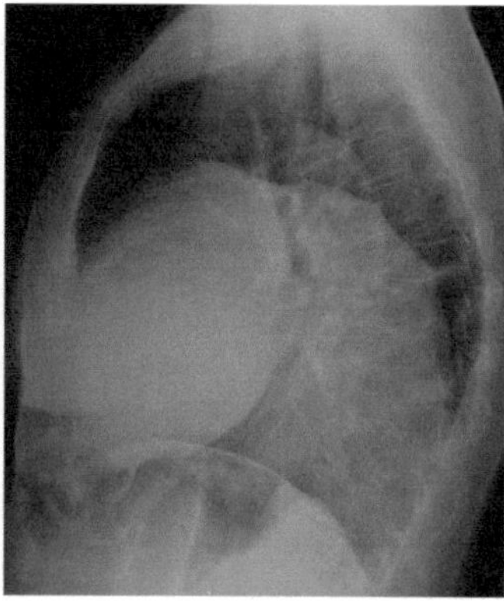

Figure 1.
Chest X-ray lateral view of a large SFTP located in the right hemithorax.

In particular, in neoplasms that reach a considerable size, areas of necrosis, haemorrhage and cystic or myxoid degeneration may be evident.

A pathognomonic radiological feature of pedunculated forms of SFTP originating from the visceral pleura is a change in shape and location of the mass during breathing or repositioning of the patient [30].

2.3.2 Computed tomography

At the computed tomography (CT) scan, SFTPs appear as a single lesion with well-defined margins arising from the chest wall (parietal pleura) or within a lung fissure (visceral pleura). They may grow up to reach remarkable dimensions, at times occupying the entire hemithorax and giving respiratory issues.

Distinctively, SFTP presents with its maximum diameter abutting the chest-wall. The lesion usually forms right or acute angles with a smooth tapering margin with the chest-wall (**Figure 2**).

Tumours arising in an interlobar fissure may be more difficult to differentiate from an intraparenchymal mass since they are surrounded by lung parenchyma.

A pathognomonic finding in pedunculated lesions is the mobility of the tumour with changes in patient position. However, this data is conditioned by the size of the tumour: the larger the tumour, the less mobile it is due to the greater number of adhesions it contracts with the surrounding tissues. It is important to evaluate the relationships with the surrounding tissues as SFTP usually presents with well-defined cleavage plans.

Another distinctive aspect of the fibrous tumour is its enhancement at the CT scan. Nearly 90% of lesions appear heterogeneous after administration of contrast, and in 75% of these a typical pattern may be recognised. Among these, the "geographic" one is the most represented. Small neoplasms tend to appear as sharp marginated masses with smooth margins, forming right or obtuse angles with the chest wall. Attenuation is homogeneous and similar to the adjacent musculature. This is a helpful feature to differentiate SFTPs from fatty lesions or saccular fluid collections. In regards to voluminous ones, they present as sharply marginated lesions with lobulated margins, creating acute angles with the chest wall. The contrast-enhanced CT evidences high attenuation of the mass due to its muscle fibres rich vascularisation, mainly and heterogeneous enhancement pattern ("geographic" the most common) with areas of necrosis, haemorrhages or cystic degeneration.

Absence of lymph nodal involvement and preservation of cleavage planes with adjacent structures provides evidence in support of the lesions' benign nature.

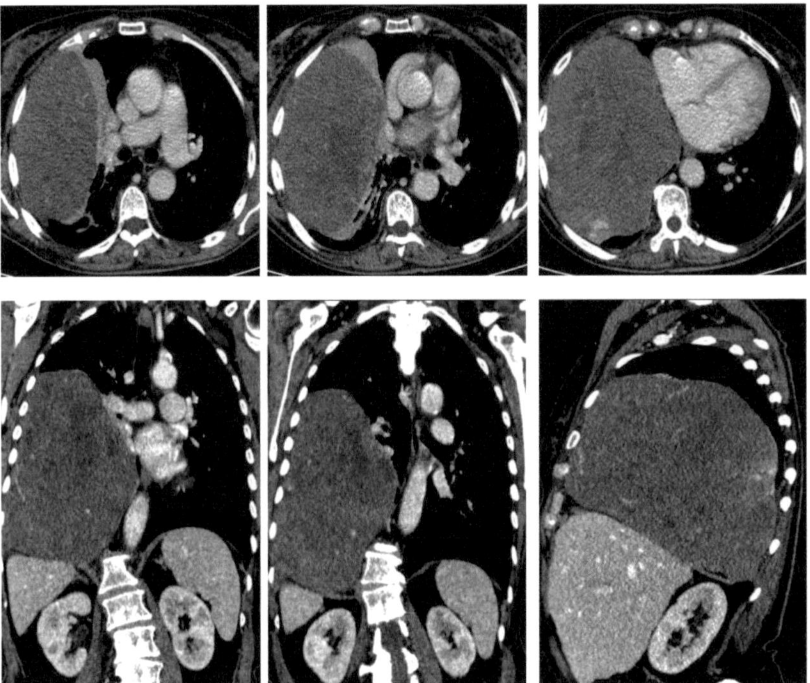

Figure 2.
Preoperative CT scan of a large SFTP in the right hemithorax.

For this reason, the presence of regional lymphadenopathy is suggestive of an alternative diagnosis.

CT therefore proves to be a very reliable imaging exam, especially when integrated with clinical and biopsy findings [30].

2.3.3 Magnetic resonance imaging

Magnetic resonance imaging (MRI) plays a limited role in the assessment of pleural disease. This exam proved to be superior to CT in studying the morphology and its relationship with the mediastinum, large vessels and diaphragm.

It is helpful in differentiating the tumour from other structures and in confirming intrathoracic localisation when the tumour abuts the diaphragm. Unfortunately, MRI patterns are quite variable in both benign and malignant SFTP [30].

2.3.4 F-18 fluoro-deoxy-glucose positron emission tomography

The role of F-18 fluoro-deoxy-glucose positron emission tomography (FDG-PET) in diagnosis of SFTP is limited and, to date, this exam is not able to discriminate between SFTP benign and malignant forms. However, it is reported its ability to identify areas of malignant transformation highlighting a focal increase of FDG uptake (SUVmax $\geq$ 3.0) within a large, otherwise benign appearing SFTP.

So, it would appear that PET scan could be useful to predict a clinically aggressive behaviour of SFTP identifying areas of malignant histology within benign SFTP [31, 32].

2.3.5 Ultrasounds

The role of ultrasound (US) in the diagnosis of SFTP is limited. These tumours, at US appear as homogeneous and hypoechoic masses, manifesting respiratory movement along-with the chest wall.

US could be useful to define the origin, thoracic vs. abdominal, of tumours which originate in close proximity with the diaphragm.

In conclusion, we can assume that it is difficult to differentiate between benign vs. malignant SFTPs based on specific radiological signs alone, albeit some radiological features are more commonly associated with malignancy (large size, central necrosis and the presence of a pleural effusion).

It is important to underline the difficulty of making a diagnosis of certainty of SFTP with the sole aid of radiological imaging, for example, as described in a case report in which a giant ectopic pleural thymoma was pre-operatively diagnosed as an SFTP due to its radiological and clinical characteristics [33].

2.4 Pathologic characteristics

SFTP is an uncommon mesenchymal tumour, characterised by typical clinical presentation and variable biological behaviour.

It was first described arising from the pleura, but similar tumours can occur in the lung, in the mediastinum (in particular in the anterior one) and in other extra-thoracic sites.

The distinctive macroscopic and histological features overlap with many other soft tissue tumours, so over the years it has been given different and very heterogeneous names such as benign mesothelioma, localised mesothelioma, solitary fibrous mesothelioma or the most famous name of hemangiopericytoma [7].

In the last decades, advances in histological, molecular and genetic research studies led to the discovery of more reliable methods of differentiating this tumour, bringing all these lesions together under the name of SFTP.

A preoperative diagnosis is usually preferable and obtained by means of a biopsy. In order to obtain as much tissue as possible for diagnosis, a radiologic guided core needle biopsy or an open incisional biopsy by an experienced surgeon is recommended [34].

2.4.1 Macroscopic description

The tumour mass is usually solitary but may also be multiple. Typically, it is well circumscribed, solid in appearance and greyish in colour, often pedunculate and with variable dimensions (often larger than 10 cm). Cystic, haemorrhagic, necrotic and calcified areas can be found.

2.4.2 Microscopic appearance

SFTP typically displays a uniform spindle cell morphology, variable cellularity—without a specific growth pattern—a marked stromal hyalinisation and branching vascular pattern. The vascular pattern is characteristic and the vessels of different numbers and sizes are so-called "staghorn" and are very similar to those described for hemangiopericytoma [35].

The cells are characterised by having a tapered nucleus and a scarce and pale cytoplasm, the nuclear atypia is often minimal. Focally, a storiform or fascicular growth pattern could be present. The stroma could rarely be myxoid. Usually, <3 mitoses can be counted for 2 mm^2, and the count of four mitoses per 2 mm^2 seems to correlate with greater aggressiveness. Necrosis is infrequent, but when present is associated with poorer prognosis (**Figure 3**).

2.4.3 Immunophenotype

Most lesions are positive for CD34 antigens but nevertheless this positivity lacks specificity in a conclusive way. Also, CD99 and Bcl2 positivity are not specific and therefore of little help. The most specific marker (>95% of cases), recently described, is STAT-6 [36] and in particular its strong and widespread nuclear reactivity (**Figure 4**). Since some de-differentiated liposarcomas can also express STAT-6, they should be kept in mind into differential diagnosis [37].

Some cases may be positive for smooth muscle actin and others for EMA (epithelial membrane agent), pancytokeratin, S100 or desmin.

2.4.4 Differential diagnosis

SFTP should be differentiated from synovial sarcoma, sarcomatoid mesothelioma, tumours of the nerve sheaths or type A Thymoma. The correct immunohistochemical reactions are necessary for a correct classification.

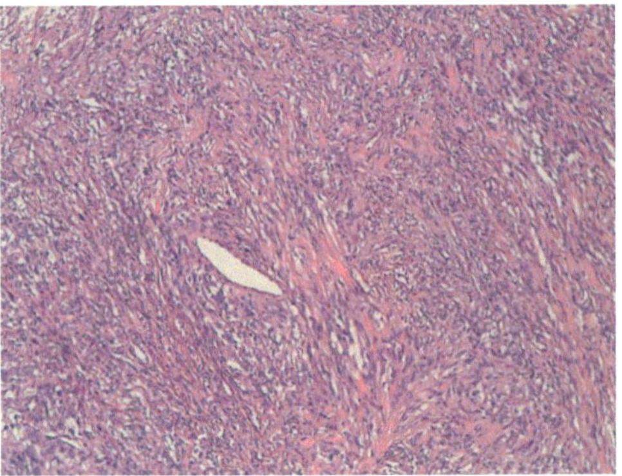

Figure 3.
Histologic features of SFTP. Morphological appearance of SFTP: typical spindle cell proliferation with low cytologic atypia (haematoxylin-eosin stain).

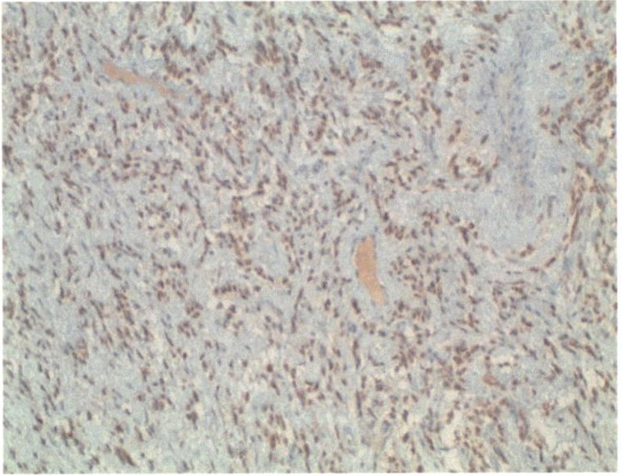

Figure 4.
Histologic features of SFTP. Immunohistochemical nuclear stain for STAT6 (IHC stain).

2.4.5 Genetic profile

SFTP harbours the gene fusion NAB2-STAT-6, which results from the intra-chromosomal inversion inv(12)(q13q13), which causes the over-expression of the protein STAT-6, found through the use of the specific antibody for the immunohistochemical reaction [12]. The over expression of IGF-2 found in some cases seems to be due to the loss of IGF-2 imprinting [38].

Telomerase reverse transcriptase (TERT) promoter mutations have been seen in 28% of SFT and are associated with high-risk pathologic characteristics and outcomes [39].

2.5 Diagnosis

The diagnosis of certainty of a SFTP is based on the histological examination of the specimen.

Usually, the first diagnostic step is a chest X-ray, performed for a different reason. The subsequent diagnostic procedure to further investigate the chest X-ray findings is a chest CT scan with contrast, which provides valuable information and orients the diagnosis towards a SFTP. As previously mentioned, this includes size and location of the tumour, the pleural origin or the presence of a stalk, areas of heterogeneity in larger lesions, an expression of the rich vascular network or intralesional haemorrhage or necrosis. These features also include the angle between the lesion and the thoracic wall which is useful when distinguishing between a pleural and a parenchymal lesion.

Larger tumours or tumours arising from the mediastinal pleura may be indistinguishable from mediastinal masses. In this case, the MRI scan is superior to the CT scan in studying the morphology and the relationship of the tumour with the mediastinum, large vessels and diaphragm. The MRI is also helpful in differentiating the tumour from other structures and better understanding margins and cleavages.

Fine needle aspiration biopsy (FNAB) is unreliable for providing a definitive diagnosis, which is mostly based on histological characteristics, as it provides insufficient tissue quantity [19], whereas a Tru-cut biopsy is more reliable. Weynand et al. reported a 100% diagnostic accuracy in determining a SFTP, using a transthoracic cutting needle [40].

2.6 Treatment

A complete surgical resection is the mainstay of the treatment of both benign and malignant SFTPs, the absence of neoplastic residual (R0) being the main prognostic factor [41].

Due to the anatomical localisation and involvement, an anatomical resection (lobectomy, bi-lobectomy or a pneumonectomy) is seldom necessary, since offers no advantages over wedge resections, for which a free margin on healthy tissue of at least 1–2 cm is recommended. In order to guarantee an adequate free margin from disease, a frozen section analysis is sometimes very useful [29]. SFTPs may occasionally require a lobectomy or a pneumonectomy when the lesion is not pedunculated but the base of implant is broad and sessile, or in case of an "inverted" tumour which grows inside the lung parenchyma.

When the tumour originates from the parietal pleura and adheres or invades the chest wall an extra-pleural dissection and a chest wall resection may be necessary [42].

Either a standard open thoracotomy or a video-assisted thoracic surgery (VATS) approach is valuable for the removal of an SFTP.

The standard open approach (posterolateral/anterolateral thoracotomy) is mandatory for patients with large tumours, multiple synchronous lesions or with obvious malignant tumours, while the VATS approach is feasible in small (up to 5.0 cm) lesions.

In case a VATS approach is preferred, it is necessary to avoid tumour dissemination using an endoscopic bag during the removal of the specimen, since contact metastases have been reported at the site of tumour extraction.

It is important to emphasise that the resection must be microscopically complete, in order to prevent late recurrence. Relapse of a benign SFTP lesion may, in fact, result in the development of a more aggressive or malignant tumour [43].

The role of adjuvant therapy in SFTP is quite limited and has not really been explored, but occasional clinical series have been reported. Suter et al. [3] studied one alive patient with no recurrence for more than 20 years after subtotal resection of the tumour followed by radiotherapy, while, Veronesi et al. [44] report the significant reduction of a recurrent fibrous tumour, not eligible for surgery, after chemotherapy with Ifosfamide and Adriamycin.

2.7 Prognosis and survival

As reported in a review [45], the overall survival of patients affected by a benign pedunculated SFTP is close to 100%. The percentage is reduced to about 92% in case of benign sessile tumour and lower in case of malignant pedunculated (85%) and malignant sessile tumour (37%). In a multicentre study, a clinicopathological staging system was presented in order to predict the clinical course or recurrences [46] with the recurrence rate distributed as reported in (**Table 2**).

Boddaert et al. [47] in their meta-analysis including over 700 patients reported a higher recurrence rate in patients with malignant histology (England's criteria), sessile morphology and incomplete resection.

Despite a recurrence after a total resection is an uncommon event, recurrences are also reported after many years, especially subsequently an incomplete resection or excision of a malignant sessile SFTP.

The most important prognostic factor seems to be a disease-free resection margin (R0); in support of this statement, Van Houdt and colleagues [46] in their series of 81 patients reported that a positive resection margin after surgery with curative intent, was correlated with local recurrence. They also reported that a high mitotic rate and tumour size >10 cm are correlated with the development of metastasis.

Recurrences may be fatal due to mediastinal invasion and superior vena cava obstruction.

In case of relapse, the primary attempt should be surgical excision, if technically and oncologically feasible, for both benign and malignant tumours.

Most recurrences occur within 24 months from surgery and are localised in the pleural cavity while distant metastasis seems to be a late event [45]. For these reasons a long-term follow-up, more than 15 years is recommended [45].

In conclusion, despite the fact that SFTPs are considered benign tumours, they may express an aggressive behaviour which leads the tumour to relapse.

Pathologically benign, pedunculated	Stage 0	2% recurrence
Pathologically benign, sessile	Stage I	8% recurrence
Malignant pathology, pedunculated	Stage II	14% recurrence
Malignant pathology, sessile	Stage III	63% recurrence

Table 2.
De Perrot staging system.

2.8 Our experience

2.8.1 Introduction

The University Unit of Thoracic Surgery of San Luigi Hospital deals with the diagnosis, treatment and follow-up of a wide range of diseases of the lung, trachea and bronchi, mediastinum and chest wall, with a specific commitment to oncological procedures by means of open and minimally invasive approaches (VATS).

Patients are referred to our Department from the outpatient clinic and through a multidisciplinary team meeting (MDT) held weekly. The present study describes a series of 64 consecutive cases, surgically treated at our Department during a 30-year period.

2.8.2 Patients and methods

This is a single-centre retrospective analysis on prospectively collected data of patients operated on for a SFTP between December 1989 and March 2019 in our Unit of Thoracic Surgery. Data was retrieved form our surgical database and variables for each patient included: gender; age at operation; symptoms; smoking history; asbestos exposure; preoperative diagnosis; CT scan; PET scan (since 2003); bronchoscopy; preoperative diagnosis; tumour origin (visceral or parietal pleura) and side (right vs. left); tumour characteristics (implant on pleura—pedunculated vs. sessile—intrapulmonary growth; size); presence of associated paraneoplastic syndromes; comorbidities (Charlson Comorbidity Index); type of resection; postoperative complications; tumour histological characteristics (Ki67%; necrosis; mitotic count).

Surgical inclusion criteria included tumour resectability, no evidences of metastases or other tumours, a good performance status (PS < 3). All patients underwent a CT scan and a preoperative bronchoscopy was performed in case of voluminous tumours. Preoperative diagnosis was attempted by means of a fine needle aspiration biopsy (FNAB) in all patients.

Postoperatively, all patients had a chest X-ray performed in post day one and after chest drain removal. Chest drains were removed when there was no air-leak detected and <250 ml of pleural fluid drained in 24/hour (**Figure 5**).

Patients' follow-up was updated by contacting all those patients known to be alive at the time of their most recent outpatient clinic attendance. Information of patients lost at follow-up was retrieved through the General Register Office. The follow-up ended on the 1 March 2019.

2.8.3 Results

A total of 64 patients were operated on for a SFTP. Twenty-eight patients were males (43.7%) and 36 females (56.3%). Mean age at surgery was 61.7 years (range 35–83 years). Thirty-one (48.4%) patients were smokers or had a history of smoking.

Thirteen patients (20.3%) were symptomatic at diagnosis with predominant symptoms being cough and chest pain. No patients reported a history of asbestos exposure (**Table 3**).

All patients underwent chest X-rays and CT scans of the chest. Positron emission tomography was performed in 12 cases (18.8%).

Fifty tumours (78.1%) were based on the visceral pleura and 14 (21.9%) arose from the parietal pleura. Thirty-five tumours (54.9%) were pedunculated while 29

(45.3%) were broad based. Among tumours arising from visceral pleura, five (7.8%) showed a prevalent intrapulmonary growth ("inverted fibroma").

The tumour was right-sided in 30 patients (46.8%) and left-side in 34 (53.2%). The lesions had a median diameter of 60 mm, the smallest tumour was 10 mm at maximum diameter and the largest was 380 mm (interquartile range: IQR-40–130 mm) (**Figure 6**).

The Charlson comorbidity index (CCI) is reported for all patients in **Table 3**.

Local excision of the pleural tumour was accomplished in 57 patients (89%). In two (3.1%) cases a wedge resection was performed and in seven patients (10.9%) an anatomical resection was required (three lobectomies, one pneumonectomy and one segmentectomy).

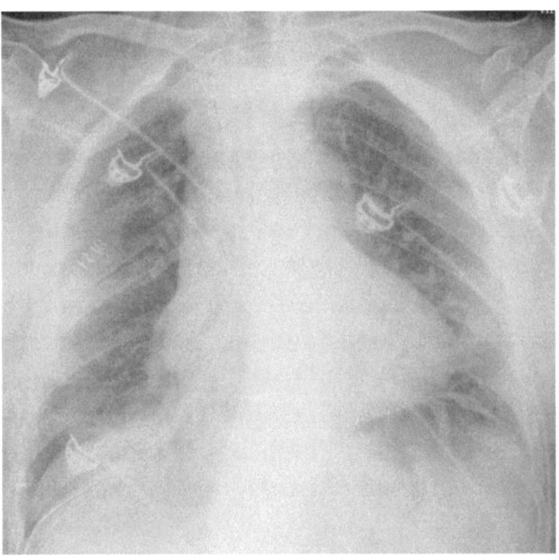

Figure 5.
Postoperative chest X-ray after radical excision of voluminous SFTP in the right hemithorax.

Age (mean, year)	61.7
Sex	
Male	28 (43.7%)
Female	36 (56.3%)
Presenting symptoms	
Cough	3
Chest pain	3
Fever	1
Dyspnoea	1
Weight loss	1
Hypoglycaemia	2
Smokers	31 (48.4%)
Charlson comorbidity index	
CCI = 0	43
CCI = 1	12
CCI = 2	7
CCI = 3	1
CCI = 4	1

Table 3.
Patient characteristics.

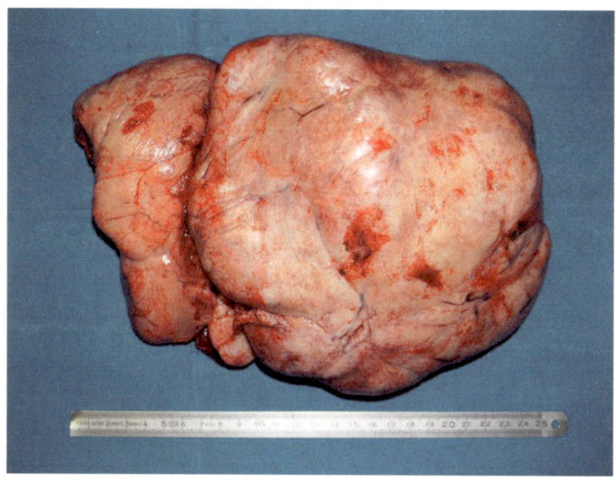

Figure 6.
Surgical specimen after a radical excision of voluminous SFTPs located in the right hemithorax.

Resection of the SFTP was performed through a thoracotomy in 51 cases (79.7%); VATS in nine cases (14.1%), and sternotomy in four cases (6.2%).

Histologically free margins were obtained in 63 cases (R0 residual disease). No patient was administered a neo-adjuvant or an adjuvant treatment.

Major postoperative complications included two atrial fibrillations, both treated with amiodarone, severe anaemia (two patients) with requirement of blood transfusions, one acute respiratory failure. Minor complications included subcutaneous emphysema (one patient), persistent air-leak from the chest drain (one patient) and atelectasis (one patient).

The histological analysis of the tumours, including Ki67% and mitosis is reported in **Table 4**.

All patients were evaluated as part of postoperative and oncological follow-up with clinical examination and chest X-ray after one and 6 months. Chest CT scan was performed every year for the first 5 years after surgery. After the first 5 years, an annual chest X-ray was recommended, or at the discretion of the general practitioner in the event of a new onset of symptoms. The annual examination is generally extended up to 15 years due to possible late onset of recurrences.

After a median follow-up of 135 months (IQR 49.2–198), 22 patients died (34.4%) and 42 are alive (65.6%). The mean disease-free interval (DFI) was 28.9 months (range: 8.7–106.1 months). In eight patients (12.5%) a single recurrence was reported while, in one patient two consecutive recurrences were identified.

Ki67	
>10%	8 (25%)
<10%	24 (75%)
N° mitosis × HPF	
>10	7 (20.6%)
<10	27 (79.4%)
Necrosis	
Present	6 (19.4%)
Absent	25 (80.6%)

Table 4.
Histology.

3. Conclusions

Solitary fibrous tumours of the pleura are rare pathological entities and are mostly discovered incidentally. Their behaviour is mostly indolent; however, some may de-dedifferentiate into malignant and aggressive tumours. Surgical resection is the mainstay treatment for SFTP, even more so in case of voluminous masses, due to compression onto lung, mediastinum and great vessels. Surgery should be carried out after a complete radiological assessment and a preoperative diagnostic attempt (FNAB), however, the diagnosis of certainty is obtained only with the definitive histological examination on surgical specimens. A long follow-up is recommended due to possible tumour recurrence.

Conflict of interest

The authors declare no conflict of interest.

Appendices and nomenclature

SFTP	solitary fibrous tumours of the pleura
HPO	hypertrophic pulmonary osteoarthropathy
IGF-2	insulin-like growth factor 2
HPF	high power fields
PDGF	platelet-derived growth factor
VEGF	vascular endothelial growth factor
CT	computed tomography
MRI	magnetic resonance imaging
FDG-PET	F-18 fluoro-deoxy-glucose positron emission tomography
US	ultrasounds
TERT	telomerase reverse transcriptase
EMA	epithelial membrane agent
FNAB	fine needle aspiration biopsy
VATS	video-assisted thoracic surgery
MDT	multidisciplinary team meeting
CCI	Charlson comorbidity index

Author details

Alberto Sandri[1*†], Alessandro Maraschi[1†], Matteo Gagliasso[1], Carlotta Cartia[1], Roberta Rapanà[1], Simona Sobrero[1], Federica Massa[2], Luisella Righi[2] and Francesco Ardissone[1]

1 Unit of Thoracic Surgery, San Luigi Gonzaga Hospital, University of Turin, Turin, Italy

2 Pathology Unit, Department of Oncology, San Luigi Gonzaga Hospital, University of Turin, Turin, Italy

*Address all correspondence to: alberto.sandri@icloud.com

† These authors equally contributed to this work.

IntechOpen

© 2019 The Author(s). Licensee IntechOpen. This chapter is distributed under the terms of the Creative Commons Attribution License (http://creativecommons.org/licenses/by/3.0), which permits unrestricted use, distribution, and reproduction in any medium, provided the original work is properly cited. CC BY

References

[1] Guinee DG, Allen TC. Primary pleural neoplasia-entities other than diffuse malignant mesothelioma. Archives of Pathology & Laboratory Medicine. 2008;**132**:1149-1170

[2] Cardillo G, Lococo F, Carleo F, et al. Solitary fibrous tumours of the pleura. Current Opinion in Pulmonary Medicine. 2012;**18**:339-346

[3] Suter M, Gebhard S, Boumghar M, et al. Localized fibrous tumours of the pleura: 15 new cases and review of the literature. European Journal of Cardio-Thoracic Surgery. 1998;**14**:453-459

[4] Magdeleinat P, Alifano M, Petino A, et al. Solitary fibrous tumours of the pleura: Clinical characteristics, surgical treatment and outcome. European Journal of Cardio-Thoracic Surgery. 2002;**21**:1087-1093

[5] Wagner E. Das tuberkelähnliche lymphadenoma (Der cytogene oder reticulirte Tuberkel). Arch Heilk. 1870;**11**:497-499

[6] Klemper P, Rabin CB. Primary neoplasm of the pleura: A report of five cases. Archives of Pathology. 1931;**11**:385-412

[7] Stout AP, Murray MR. Hemangiopericytoma: A vascular tumour featuring Zimmerman's pericytes. Annals of Surgery. 1942;**116**:26-33

[8] Hernandez FJ, Hernandez BB. Localized fibrous tumours of the pleura: A light and electron microscopic study. Cancer. 1974;**34**:1667-1674

[9] Al-Azzi M, Thurlow NP, Corrin B. Pleural mesothelioma of connective tissue type, localized fibrous tumour of the pleura, and reactive submesothelial hyperplasia: An immunohisto-chemical comparison. The Journal of Pathology. 1989;**158**:41-44

[10] Markku M. Chapter 12: Solitary fibrous tumour, hemangiopericytoma, and related tumours. In: Mettinen M, editor. Modern Soft Tissue Pathology: Tumours and Non-Neoplastic Conditions. New York: Cambridge University Press; 2010. p. 335

[11] Demicco EG, Park MS, Araujo DM, Fox PS, Bassetti RL, Pollock RE, et al. Solitary fibrous tumour. A clinicopathological study of 110 cases and proposed risk assessment model. Modern Pathology. 2012;**25**(9):1298-1306

[12] Robinson DR, Wu YM, Kalyana-Sundaram S, et al. Identification of recurrent NAB2-STAT6 gene fusions in solitary fibrous tumourby integrative sequencing. Nature Genetics. 2013;**45**:180-185

[13] Chmielecki J, Crago AM, Rosenberg M, et al. Whole-exome sequencing indentifies a recurrent NAB2-STAT6 fusion in solitary fibrous tumours. Nature Genetics. 2013;**45**:131-132

[14] Sung SH, Chang JW, Kim J, et al. Solitary fibrous tumours of the pleura: Surgical outcome and clinical course. The Annals of Thoracic Surgery. 2005;**79**:303-307

[15] Okike N, Bernatz PE, Woolner LB. Localized mesothelioma of the pleura: Benign and malignant variants. The Journal of Thoracic and Cardiovascular Surgery. 1978;**75**:363-361

[16] Rosado-de-Christenson ML, Abbott GF, McAdams HP, et al. Localized fibrous tumours of the pleura. Radiographics. 2003;**23**:759-783

[17] Harrison RI, McCaughan BC. Malignancy in a massive localized fibrous tumour of the pleura. Australian and New Zealand Journal of Surgery. 1992;**62**:311-313

[18] England DM, Hochholzer L, McCarthy MJ. Localized benign and malignant fibrous tumours of the pleura. A clinicopathologic review of 223 cases. The American Journal of Surgical Pathology. 1989;**13**:640-658

[19] Robinson LA. Solitary fibrous tumours of the pleura. Cancer Control. 2006;**13**:264-269

[20] Localized fibrous tumours of the pleura. In: Shields, General Thoracic Surgery. 8th ed. Philadelphia: Wolters Kluwer; 2019

[21] Marie P. De l'osteo-arthropatie hypertrophiante pneumique. La Revue de Médecine Paris. 1890;**10**:1-36

[22] von Bamberger E. Veränderungen der röhrenknochen bei bronchiektasie. Wiener Klinische Wochenschrift. 1889;**2**:226

[23] Tachibana I, Gehi D, Rubin CD. Treatment of hypertrophic osteoarthropaty with underlying pulmonary adenocarcinoma using zoledronic acid. Journal of Clinical Rheumatology. 2015;**21**:333-334

[24] Hojo S, Fujita J, Yamadori I, et al. Hepatocyte growth factor and digital clubbing. Internal Medicine. 1997;**36**:44-46

[25] Doege KW. Fibrosarcoma of the mediastinum. Annals of Surgery. 1930;**92**:955-960

[26] Potter RP. Intrathoracic tumours. Radiology. 1930;**14**:60-62

[27] Meng W, Zhu HH, Li H, Wang G, Wei D, Feng X. Solitary fibrous tumours of the pleura with Doege-Potter syndrome: A case report and three-decade review of the literature. BMC Research Notes. 2014;7:515

[28] de Groot JW, Rikhof B, van Doorn J, et al. Non-islet cell tumour-induced hypoglycaemia: A review of the literature including two new cases. Endocrine-Related Cancer. 2007;**14**(14):979-993

[29] de Perrot M, Fischer S, Brundler MA, et al. Solitary fibrous tumours of the pleura. The Annals of Thoracic Surgery. 2002;**74**:285-293

[30] Cardinale L, Allasia M, Ardissone F, Borasio P, Familiari U, Lausi P, et al. CT features of solitary fibrous tumour of the pleura: Experience in 26 patients. La Radiologia Medica. 2006;**111**:640-650

[31] Hara M, Kume M, Oshima H, et al. F-18 FDG uptae in a malignant localized fibrous tumour of the pleura. Journal of Thoracic Imaging. 2005;**20**(2):118-119

[32] Dong A, Zuo C, Wang Y, et al. Enhanced CT and FDG PET/CT in malignant solitary fibrous tumour of the lung. Clinical Nuclear Medicine. 2014;**39**:488-491

[33] Filosso PL, Delsedime L, Cristofori RC, Sandri A. Ectopic pleural thymoma mimicking a giant solitary fibrous tumour of the pleura. Interactive Cardiovascular and Thoracic Surgery. 2012;**15**(5):930-932

[34] Weynand B, Noel H, Goncette L, et al. Solitary fibrous tumour of the pleura: A report of five cases diagnosed by transthoracic cutting needle biopsy. Chest. 1997;**112**:1424-1428

[35] Gold JS, Antonescu CR, Hajdu C, et al. Clinicopathologic correlates of solitary fibrous tumours. Cancer. 2002;**94**:1057-1068

[36] Yoshida A, Tsuta K, Ohno M, et al. STAT6 immunohistochemistry is helpful in the diagnosis of solitary fibrous tumours. The American Journal of Surgical Pathology. 2014;**38**:552-559

[37] Doyle LA, Vivero M, Fletcher CDM, et al. Nuclear expression of STAT6

distinguishes solitary fibrous tumour from histologic mimics. Modern Pathology. 2014;**27**:390-395

[38] Hajdu M, Singer S, Maki RG, et al. IGF2 over-expression in SFT is independent of anatomical location and is related to loss of imprinting. The Journal of Pathology. 2010;**221**:300-301

[39] Bahrami A, Lee S, Schaefer IM, et al. TERT promoter mutations and prognosis in solitary fibrous tumour. Modern Pathology. 2016;**29**:1511-1522

[40] Weynand B, Collard P, Galant C. Cytopathological features of solitary fibrous tumour of the pleura: A study of 5 cases. Diagnostic Cytopathology. 1998;**18**:118-124

[41] Rena O, Filosso PL, Papalia E, et al. Solitary fibrous tumour of the pleura: Surgical treatment. European Journal of Cardio-Thoracic Surgery. 2001;**19**:185-189

[42] Magdaleinat P, Alifano M, Petino A, et al. Solitary fibrous tumour of the pleura: Clinical characteristics, surgical treatment and outcome. European Journal of Cardio-Thoracic Surgery. 2002;**21**:1087-1093

[43] Mashes B, Clelland C, Ratnatunga C. Recurrent localized fibrous tumour fo the pleura. The Annals of Thoracic Surgery. 2006;**82**:342-345

[44] Veronesi G, Spaggiari L, Mazzarol G, et al. Huge malignant localized fibrous tumour of the pleura. The Journal of Cardiovascular Surgery. 2000;**41**:781-784

[45] de Perrot M, Kurt AM, Robert JH, et al. Clinical behavior of solitary fibrous tumours of the pleura. The Annals of Thoracic Surgery. 1999;**67**:1456-1459

[46] van Houdt WJ, Westerveld CM, Vrijenhoek JE, et al. Prognosis of solitary fibrous tumours: A multicenter study. Annals of Surgical Oncology. 2013;**20**:4090-4095

[47] Boddaert G, Guiraudet P, Grand B, et al. Solitary fibrous tumours of the pleura: A poorly defined malignancy profile. The Annals of Thoracic Surgery. 2015;**99**:1025-1031